Skills Training in Communication and Related Topics Part 1

Skills Training in Communication and Related Topics Part 1

Dealing with conflict and change

ELLEN J BELZER

MPA

President, Belzer Seminars and Consulting,
Missouri, USA

Radcliffe Publishing
Oxford • New York

Radcliffe Publishing Ltd
18 Marcham Road
Abingdon
Oxon OX14 1AA
United Kingdom

www.radcliffe-oxford.com
Electronic catalogue and worldwide online ordering facility.

British Library Cataloguing in Publication Data

A catalogue record for this book is available from the British Library.

ISBN-13: 978 1 84619 277 7

Typeset by Pindar NZ, Auckland, New Zealand
Printed and bound by Cadmus Communications, USA

Contents

BY ACTIVITY

CONFLICT MANAGEMENT

NEGOTIATION – BARGAINING SKILLS

Session openers

Case studies

Role-play exercises

DEALING WITH DIFFICULT COLLEAGUES

Session openers

Case studies

DIFFICULT CONVERSATIONS

COMMUNICATING IN CRISIS SITUATIONS

DEALING WITH ORGANIZATIONAL CHANGE

The *Skills Training* series is dedicated to the memory of my dear friend and mentor,
R Michael Miller.

About the author

Ellen J Belzer, MPA, is president of Belzer Seminars and Consulting, LLC, a Kansas City based company specializing in negotiation, management, and communication programs and services for health care professionals. For more than 20 years, her seminars have been conducted for many thousands of healthcare professionals throughout the United States. In addition to serving as a professional mediator and organizational consultant, she frequently facilitates strategic planning and brainstorming sessions for public and private sector health care organizations. Prior to starting her seminar and consulting practice in 1986, she was an executive at a national medical specialty society for 12 years where she received a broad background in medical socioeconomics.

Ellen currently serves on the adjunct faculty of the dispute resolution programs at Baker University and Johnson County Community College, both in Overland Park, Kansas. She previously served as a communications instructor at Avila University in Kansas City, Missouri, and also taught negotiation and leadership development courses for the University of Kansas. She received her BA degree from Northwestern University in Evanston, Illinois, and her Master of Public Administration degree from the University of Missouri at Kansas City. She received additional training in negotiation from intensive programs at several leading universities in the United States.

Introduction

As numerous communications texts point out, we tend to remember 10% of what we read, 20% of what we hear, 30% of what we see, 50% of what we see and hear, 70% of what we say, and 90% of what we say and do. What could be a stronger argument for using teaching methods that *actively* involve participants?

Just as **learning by doing** is extremely helpful for teaching clinical procedures, it is especially helpful when teaching communication and related topics. First you explain and demonstrate the strategies; then participants try them out. Demonstrations, games, case study discussions, role plays, and other group involvement activities are fun and engaging and, more importantly, they enable learners to immediately process what they've learned. Through experiential exercises, people learn from their successes and missteps in a safe environment. They also learn from the skillful critiques of their colleagues as well as from mentors, faculty members, and leaders of their health care teams.

With packed curricula in most health care training institutions and hectic schedules in busy practices and administrative offices, there may not be much time left for teaching communication and related topics. Even though clinical topics must necessarily take precedence, that doesn't mean that communication and related topics can be ignored. After all, communication relates to practically everything health care professionals do. Whether discussing a treatment plan with a patient, conferring with a colleague, making a referral, negotiating with a managed care organization, discussing new policies in a staff meeting, supervising an employee, or dealing with a conflict, effective communication skills are critical. Moreover, quality communication contributes to smoother running practices, better care and services, greater efficiencies, fewer unhealthy conflicts, more satisfied staff and patients, and an improved ability to meet the challenges of an evolving and increasingly complex health care environment.

The three volumes of *Skills Training in Communication and Related Topics* are intended for practice leaders, hospital leaders, and public health professionals who want to help health care professionals upgrade their skills, and *especially* for faculty members who teach students and residents. The series is designed for use in virtually any training situation, whether you're conducting an in-service, a noon conference, a workshop, a seminar, or other forms of more extended training. This book (Part 1) is devoted to topics that will enable your trainees to deal more effectively with conflict, difficult behaviors, and other complex situations. Part 2 contains training exercises on communicating with patients, colleagues, and communities, and Part 3 addresses leadership/management and organizational skills.

I've developed this series on the basis of two premises: that you'll *find* time to teach communication and related subjects to health care professionals and that you'll *save* time by utilizing the activities provided to you. The exercises mapped out for you in these books take into consideration your limited training time for non-clinical topics. Some exercises take minutes while others take an hour or more, so you can select the exercises that would work best in the amount of time you have available.

In the future, I hope there will be new editions of this series so that I can incorporate your ideas for other training activities. If you'd like to contribute to new editions, please let me hear from you!

Ellen J Belzer, MPA
Email: ellen@healthcarecollaborator.com or
belzersc@juno.com
Website: www.belzerseminars.com

Acknowledgments

Many people deserve special thanks for their contributions to this book. First, many thanks to Angie Callison for suggesting that I make use of the many boxes of training exercises I've been amassing for decades, and to Patty Swyden Sullivan who provided invaluable editing assistance and suggestions.

I owe an enormous debt to the superb faculty of the Providence Family Medicine Residency in Southfield, Michigan, for their review of many of the physician-related case studies and role plays to ensure their relevance and accuracy. Thank you to Karen Mitchell, MD, Program Director, and faculty members (in alphabetical order): Robert Brummeler, MD, Gary G Otsuji, MD, Jill Schneiderhan, MD, and Susan C Zeltzer, MD.

For their review of numerous public health-related cases and role plays, I extend my deepest thanks to Dr. Donna Petersen, Dean of the College of Public Health at the University of South Florida and Director of the Maternal and Child Health Leadership Skills Institute, and Cathy Chadwick, MPH, the Institute's Project Coordinator.

Because numerous exercises in this book were originally published in *The Healthcare Collaborator* (HCC), an online newsletter that I published from 2000–03, I extend my thanks to members of the HCC Board of Advisors (in alphabetical order): Bruce Bagley, MD; Helen H Baker, PhD, MBA; Stephen Brunton, MD; Angeline Bushy, PhD, RN, CS, FAAN; Gregory Carroll, PhD; Kevin Fickenscher, MD; Steven P Geiermann, DDS; Romeo J Guerra, MA; Charlotte L Hardt, BSN, MSHA; Molly Hartshorn, MSHP, CMPE; A Clinton MacKinney, MD, MS; Ross P Marine, DHL, MHA; Lee N Newcomer, MD; Dave Palm, PhD; Patrick L Patterson; Michael P Rosenthal, MD; Roger A Sherwood; and Donna M Williams. Extra thanks are due to two of these advisors, Steven P Geiermann, DDS, and Roger A Sherwood, for their many extra hours of careful reviews, editing assistance, and sage advice. Thank you, Steve and Roger.

A world of thanks is also due to Gillian Nineham of Radcliffe Publishing, for believing in this project and making this series possible, to Andrea Hargreaves, Ollie Judkins and other valued members of Radcliffe's editorial staff for their outstanding work, and to Jane Gadd and the production team at Pindar NZ for their superb production and Ruth Blaikie for her excellent editing.

In regard to everyone who helped: Whatever you liked most about this book is because of them; any mistakes are entirely mine!

Last but not least, thanks to the many thousands of participants in my training programs and mediations over the past 20-plus years that provided the field testing for many of the training tools you'll find in this book as well as in Parts 2 and 3. As you utilize the exercises herein to enhance the communication skills and competencies of your learners, I hope you'll give your trainees the same advice I repeatedly give to mine: "Have fun while you're learning!" -- EJB

Using this book

Let's begin by addressing some of the questions you may have about using the training material in this book.

Can I make copies of the handout material provided in this book?
Yes! Handouts for participants are contained on separate pages following the instructions. The handout material is also available at www.radcliffe-oxford.com/trainingtools

Can I modify the exercises?
If you don't want to use these exact exercises, feel free to modify them to fit your particular training needs. Even if you don't use the exercises in this book, it is hoped that you can get ideas from them.

As a word of caution, however, don't be too quick to make changes that would homogenize the role-play exercises by changing the characters to persons in your field alone. If some learners balk at the idea of playing the role of someone from a different profession or discipline, encourage them to stretch. There's a great deal of learning in trying to see things from someone else's window on the world.

Other than the exercises, what should be the content of the training sessions?
Begin each session with a brief lecture on the topic you're teaching so that learners will be able to practice new strategies. While this book provides activities that will enliven your training, your course design and content is up to you. Refer to the reading list at the end of the book for resource material.

What are the special features of this book?
Three matrices at the end of this book will help you determine which exercises best meet your specific training needs. Matrix 1 shows which exercises are recommended for each training topic; Matrix 2 identifies which exercises are best for persons in various types of health professions; and Matrix 3 identifies each exercise by length so that you can select those that best fit into your available time slots.

The appendices also contain tips for trainers, suggestions on managing the critique sessions that you will conduct after the exercises, and a sampling of quotations about each of the suggested training topics to add pizzazz to your training programs.

How accurate are the suggested training times?
Times have been estimated for groups of 15 or fewer. For training programs involving more participants, add extra time for group reporting and discussions.

Definitions

ICEBREAKERS
These are warm-up exercises that introduce the topic, create interest in the subject matter, and set the stage for group involvement.

INTRODUCTORY DISCUSSIONS
Like icebreakers, these discussions are intended to help participants address a specific aspect of the topic while getting them engaged in group process.

SELF-TESTS
These tests help to make the training more individualized and enable trainees to understand their own traits and tendencies regarding the subject matter.

WORKSHEETS
After participants write their responses to the questions on these forms, the facilitator leads a group discussion about their responses. The purpose is to help learners focus on the concepts being taught.

CASE STUDIES
Some case studies are more detailed than others, but all are brief enough to process in relatively short spans of time. After participants have read the cases, ask them to analyze them and make recommendations either in small-group or all-group discussions. If you decide to break into small groups, ask a representative from each to report their findings to the group as a whole. If you'd prefer, you can convert the case studies into role plays by assigning participants to act as each of the characters.

ROLE-PLAY EXERCISES
These exercises are designed for groups of two, three, four, or five, as each role play requires. If there are extra persons, assign them to double in a role with another character or ask them to serve as observers.

Some role-play exercises have a separate page of "General Instructions" (to distribute to everyone), followed by separate "Confidential Instructions" (to distribute to persons playing each role). Other role-play exercises use character roles only and do not have separate General Instructions. For ease of distribution, make copies of each character role on a different color paper.

After instructions are distributed, instruct participants to act out the scene from their character's viewpoint. Tell participants they may change their behaviors or positions only if the points raised by other characters would cause them to do so in a real-life situation. If more details are needed in some of the shorter role-play exercises, advise participants that they can embellish the "facts" of the cases as long as their points are consistent with their assigned roles.

PRACTICE EXERCISES

These are brief exercises that allow participants to refine their skills by immediately applying new strategies.

DEBRIEFING

An essential part of the training, this is a facilitated discussion following each activity in which participants dissect the training activity and analyze the quality of their responses. It is also a perfect time for you to drive home the key teaching points. Discussion questions are provided to help you facilitate this portion of the session.

> Note: While some names of characters in the case studies and role-play exercises have been modeled after well-known persons or fictitious characters, this has been done for the amusement of readers (and the author), and any resemblance to real persons, living or dead, is entirely coincidental. The case studies and role plays are either fictitious or are composites of numerous situations.

Conflict management

Five professional goals

TYPE: Icebreaker

ESTIMATED TRAINING TIME: 15 minutes

THEMES: Conflict management, negotiation

OBJECTIVES:
➡ to show the tendency to view conflict as a win-lose situation;
➡ to demonstrate the win-win approach to conflict management and negotiation.

MATERIALS NEEDED: None

PROCEDURE:
Tell the group that they will do a brief exercise to illustrate the best way to resolve conflict or negotiate, depending on the topic of your training session. Ask the group:

> "Please think of five professional goals that you would like to reach by the end of the year."

Tell them they don't have to actually write down their goals; they just need to assume that they each have five goals to reach. Then ask each participant to choose a partner.

After the pairings, ask for a volunteer to demonstrate how the exercise will work. When the volunteer comes to the front of the room, demonstrate an arm-wrestling position, but *without* using the term "arm-wrestling," since that might affect how participants approach this task. Ask the volunteer to put his/her right arm in the same position.

Then guide the volunteer through the exercise:

> "Every time I get Dr. Smith's arm down on the other side of the table, I get one of my goals met. Every time Dr. Smith gets my arm down to the other side of the table, she gets one of her goals met. You will have 30 seconds to complete the exercise and meet your five goals."

As the volunteer is reseated, tell participants that there are three rules:
1 No verbal communication is allowed until the exercise is completed.
2 You will only have 30 seconds to reach your goals.
3 No one can hurt anyone else!

Ask for any questions about the exercise; then say, "Please begin."

DEBRIEFING:

After the 30-second time limit, begin the debriefing by asking for a show of hands:

> "How many of you did not meet any of your goals? One goal? Two? Three? Four? Five?"

Illustrate the difference between those who did not meet any of their goals and those who achieved all of them. Those who got only a few goals met were most likely in a tug-of-war, with each party trying to force the other. Those who got most or all of their goals met most likely took turns getting each other's arms down, thus enabling one another to fulfill all of their needs.

Then ask the following questions:

1 In what ways was this exercise a metaphor for conflict management and negotiation in the workplace?

2 When attempting to influence or persuade colleagues or patients, what does this exercise tell us about communicating *with* them rather than *at* them?

3 Even though those who used force may have gotten at least some of their immediate needs met, what would be the long-term effect of using this approach when dealing with colleagues?

4 If you got all five of your goals met, what factors contributed to your success? What is the lesson here about the benefits of meeting the other party's needs as well as your own? (Point out that those who met more than the five goals they were asked to obtain did an especially good job; when you're on a roll in problem-solving, it pays to keep going!)

Point out that "win-win" outcomes are those in which both parties get all, most, or at least some, of their major needs met. When both parties work *with* one another, meeting the five goals (or more) within 30 seconds is an easy matter. But when both parties only consider their own needs and view the conflict as an "I win-you lose" contest, the conflict turns into a power struggle. In such cases, achieving any of the goals becomes an arduous and sometimes painful task.

Dissecting a common conflict

TYPE: Introductory discussion

ESTIMATED TRAINING TIME: 15 minutes

THEME: Conflict management

OBJECTIVES:

➡ to explore the root causes of a common conflict;

➡ to understand that conflicts frequently have structural causes (e.g. outdated or unclear organizational policies or procedures, etc.), despite the common tendency to blame individuals;

➡ to help participants shift gears from problem identification to a focus on solutions.

MATERIALS NEEDED: Flip chart (optional)

PROCEDURE:

First, ask the group to identify the types of disputes that seem to be recurring most frequently in your health care setting.

Next, select the most prevalent type of conflict and ask delving questions to get to its root. For issues identified as "people problems," ask the group to identify aspects of the health care organization that could have contributed to the problem behaviors. For example, "Have any organizational policies or job stresses contributed to people's negative behaviors? What changes in workplace procedures may have been factors?" Write the root causes on a flip chart if you're using one.

Ask the group to brainstorm on possible solutions. Remind the group to develop solutions that address each of the root causes they have identified.

DEBRIEFING:

1 What are the key lessons you have gleaned from this discussion?

2 How would the suggested solutions have differed if we hadn't explored the true nature of the conflict first?

3 How can the solutions that were suggested during our brainstorming be applied to our health care setting? Which would work best?

Training Tool #3

What are your hot buttons?

TYPE: Introductory discussion

ESTIMATED TRAINING TIME: 15 minutes

THEMES: Conflict management, negotiation, difficult colleagues, difficult conversations, communicating in crisis situations, organizational change, emotional intelligence

OBJECTIVES:

➡ to identify emotional triggers that can result in negative reactions, causing conflicts to develop or escalate;

➡ to ascertain ways to control negative reactions.

MATERIALS NEEDED: Flip chart (optional)

PROCEDURE:

Define "hot button" as a verbal or nonverbal trigger that evokes an emotional response and can either lead you into conflict or cause a conflict to escalate or worsen. Also point out that when your hot button is pressed, you normally "tune out" and no longer listen to the speaker.

Ask group members to discuss the types of comments or behaviors that tend to press their hot buttons during conflicts. (Examples might include people who say, "You have failed to realize . . .," referring to nurses as "support staff," arrogant behaviors, colleagues who come to work late, etc.) If desired, list these responses on a flip chart.

DEBRIEFING:

1 In answering these questions, did you notice that what is a "hot button" to one person isn't always as disturbing to someone else?

2 What are your likely reactions when people press your "hot button"?

3 When your "hot buttons" are pressed and you do nothing to neutralize your reaction, how does that affect your ability to deal with conflict?

4 What strategies work best for controlling negative first reactions?

The need to
think through our
responses in conflict
situations

First reactions

TYPE: Introductory discussion

ESTIMATED TRAINING TIME: 15 minutes

THEMES: Conflict management, negotiation, difficult colleagues, difficult conversations, communicating in crisis situations, organizational change, emotional intelligence

OBJECTIVES:
- to show that people's first reaction to negative comments or behaviors is often to respond in kind with another negative response;
- to demonstrate that while negative tit-for-tat responses are normal human reactions, we need to resist these impulses because they usually worsen the conflict rather than lead to its resolution.

MATERIALS NEEDED: Flip chart (optional)

PROCEDURE:
Ask participants these questions:

> "When someone yells at you, what is your first usual reaction?" (Most will say, "Yell back.")

> "When you feel like someone is attacking you, what do you want to do?" ("Attack them back.")

> "What is your first reaction when someone ignores you?" ("Ignore them even more!")

DEBRIEFING:
1 What are the effects of responding to negative behaviors by relying on your first negative reaction?" (Write responses on a flip chart if you're using one.)
2 What are some possible reasons for our first response usually being negative, i.e. one that works against us?
3 What can we do to avoid relying on our first negative response?

Characteristics of healthy vs unhealthy conflict

TYPE: Worksheet

ESTIMATED TRAINING TIME: 15 minutes

THEME: Conflict management

OBJECTIVES:

➥ to illustrate the differences between conflicts that are handled in a healthy (positive) way versus those that are handled in an unhealthy (negative) way;

➥ to point out the benefits of healthy conflict to the health care team and organization, and why it's important to avoid unhealthy conflict.

MATERIALS NEEDED: A copy of the worksheet on the next page for each participant; prizes are optional.

PROCEDURE:

Distribute copies of the worksheet and tell the group that they will have five minutes to jot down the characteristics of healthy conflict (ways of handling conflicts that are beneficial to health care teams and organizations) versus unhealthy conflict (ways of handling conflicts that are deleterious to health care teams and organizations). Consider offering a small prize to the person who identifies the most characteristics.

DEBRIEFING:

1 What are the key ways that healthy conflict differs from unhealthy conflict?
2 What are the advantages of a healthy conflict to the health care team? To the health care organization?
3 What are the effects of unhealthy conflicts on the workplace?
4 How can you avoid unhealthy conflicts in the first place?

Worksheet

What are the characteristics of healthy and unhealthy conflicts in health care settings?

HEALTHY CONFLICT	UNHEALTHY CONFLICT

The effects of
regarding conflict in
a negative light

Word association and conflict

TYPE: Worksheet

ESTIMATED TRAINING TIME: 15 minutes

THEME: Conflict management

OBJECTIVES:

➡ to demonstrate our human tendency to view conflict in a negative light;

➡ to show that when conflict is viewed as an opportunity, there are likely to be many benefits to those involved as well as to the health care team and the organization.

MATERIALS NEEDED: A copy of the worksheet on the next page for each participant; prizes are optional.

PROCEDURE:

Tell the group that they will have to work fast, as they only have three minutes to free associate whatever words occur to them when they think of the word "conflict." (Consider offering a small prize to the person who lists the most responses in the three-minute period.)

DEBRIEFING:

1 How many words did you free associate with the word "conflict"? Of those, how many were negative versus positive?

2 How many regarded conflict as an opportunity – or in other positive terms?

3 How does your attitude toward conflict affect the way you are likely to manage it?

WORKSHEET

When I think of *conflict*, the words that come to mind are . . .

1 _____

2 _____

3 _____

4 _____

5 _____

6 _____

7 _____

8 _____

9 _____

10 _____

11 _____

12 _____

13 _____

14 _____

15 _____

Turf wars

TYPE: Case study

ESTIMATED TRAINING TIME: 30 minutes

THEMES: Conflict management, negotiation, difficult colleagues

OBJECTIVES:
➡ to understand that parties involved in a conflict can each have valid points;
➡ to identify ways to convert positions into mutual interests;
➡ to raise awareness about turf issues in health care settings.

MATERIALS NEEDED: Copies of the case study on the next page for all participants

PROCEDURE:
Provide an overview about turf battles in health care settings and point out that while some of the issues involve territoriality, there can also be legitimate issues that need to be addressed between departments, divisions, units, or other groups of health care professionals.

Distribute copies of the case study and give the group a minute or so to read it. For a large group, divide participants into small groups of three to five persons each and ask each group to report on their analysis and recommendations to the group as a whole after a 10–15 minute discussion.

DEBRIEFING:
1 What are the underlying issues in this dispute?
2 Does Dr. Burns have a valid point, given that radiology provides services to all other specialties as well as to family medicine? Does Dr. Pierce have valid needs as well?
3 What should Dr. Pierce say or do differently in order to ensure that the Department of Family Medicine's needs are met? How should Dr. Burns communicate differently at their upcoming meeting?
4 How would you suggest that this issue be resolved?
5 How do turf wars within health care organizations affect others – aside from those directly involved?

CASE STUDY: TURF WARS

Dr. Ben Pierce, Chair of the Department of Family Medicine, has recently "had words" with the radiology department for not providing services on a timely basis. The Chair of the Department of Radiology, Dr. Franklin Burns, says that he doesn't take orders from the family medicine department and that other departments within the medical center have equally pressing needs.

The discussions between Drs. Pierce and Burns have become so acrimonious that the medical center's CEO, Ms. Margaret Hooligan, decided to step in. She told the radiology chair to be more cooperative and asked the family medicine chair to be less aggressive. She also asked both department chairs to meet once again to work out their differences. She noted that she planned to attend that meeting as well, and that she expected them to come armed with possible solutions.

Dr. Pierce is looking forward to this meeting because he believes that the family medicine department is still not getting optimal service from radiology. He believes that the radiology department is mismanaged. Because radiology is fully staffed now – having recently recruited two new radiologists who came to the medical center just in the past week – he cannot see why it is taking so long to get patients tested, and why there's such a long delay getting reports on the results from MRIs and ultrasounds.

Dr. Burns is also looking forward to this meeting as he plans to more forcefully make his point that radiology serves the entire medical center – not just family medicine. He resents implications that his department isn't well-managed; the unusually high influx of patient admissions during recent months has been responsible for some, if not most, of the current backlog. He also wants to point out that there have been an unusually high number of requests to work high-risk patients into the schedule.

Generational conflict

TYPE: Case study

ESTIMATED TRAINING TIME: 30 minutes

THEME: Conflict management

OBJECTIVES:

➡ to explore the perspectives and tendencies of employees in different age groups that can lead to conflict in health care organizations;

➡ to identify ways to bridge generational conflicts among older and younger members of the health care team.

MATERIALS NEEDED: Copies of the case study on the following pages for all participants

PROCEDURE:

To begin, ask: "Do you believe that personnel in our health care organization view things differently depending on their age?" Most responses will be "yes," or "it depends on the issue," but some will say that differences are individualized and efforts should be made to avoid stereotyping. Then ask, "In what ways, if at all, do generational differences contribute to conflict in our organization?"

Distribute copies of the case study on Generational Conflict to all participants and give the group about five minutes for review.

DEBRIEFING:

1 What is your assumption about the age range or generation of Dorothy, Blanche, Rose, and Sophia? What is the likely generation of BeBe and Johnny?
2 What are the differences between the characters in these two scenes?
3 Given that the characters in both scenes seem uncomfortable in their working relationships, what can they do to bridge this gap and work together more effectively as a team?
4 What are the benefits of developing a better understanding of generational differences?
5 What are the implications of generational differences for health care leaders and managers?

CASE STUDY: GENERATIONAL CONFLICT

While having lunch in the New Age Medical Center's cafeteria, a group of colleagues discussed some of the frustrations they had recently experienced with other staff members.

"I must be getting old," said Dorothy Zorback, Director of Medical Records. "We've been hiring so many of these younger kids, right out of college or health professions' training, and I just don't understand their work ethic."

"What's happening?" Blanche Dubois asked.

"Well, every time I try to give them advice and tell them the way things work around here, they don't want to listen," Dorothy replied. "They have no respect for authority. *We* were never like that."

"I know what you mean!" chimed in Rose Myland. "These young ones don't realize we've been here for our entire careers and that we do know a thing or two!"

"What's worse is that they keep telling me what needs to be done differently!" Dorothy said.

"Like what?" Rose inquired.

"Well, they want shorter hours. One said, 'I work to live – I don't live to work.' Do you believe that? And they're always on the computer. Plus, they barely know the ropes here, yet they want me to switch to different software."

Blanche grimaced. "I hate computers. Just when I'm learning one type of program, they give me another kind. I just can't seem to wrap my brain around this stuff."

Sophia Perpetuallo nodded. "I know what you mean, Blanche. Not to mention that these kids keep sending emails and text messages. Whatever happened to good old face-to-face communication?"

* * *

Across the room, Frances (BeBe) Holmes, LPN, is telling a friend about a dilemma she is facing. "I'm not having a good day," said BeBe. "Our nursing supervisor just had a meeting with us about her new rules. No tardiness or she'll write us up. She wants to be called 'Mrs. Schumacher,' never by her first name. Plus, she wants us to fill out several more detailed forms to put into patient charts . . . as if we have extra time on our hands!"

"Have you tried to talk with her?" asked Johnny Palace, a fourth-year medical student.

"Only when I asked if I could work a shorter shift," BeBe replied. "She said I'm lucky to have this work and that I didn't realize how hard things used to be in the old days."

"I guess she *would* think that," Johnny said. "I've already had several run-ins with Mrs. Schumacher myself. She thinks she's right about everything. I just wish that when she's wrong, she'd say she's wrong."

BeBe sighed. "I feel like I'm being micromanaged these days. No wonder I've been feeling like people are always trying to put me in a corner."

Not my job

TYPE: Case study

ESTIMATED TRAINING TIME: 30 minutes

THEMES: Conflict management, negotiation, difficult colleagues

OBJECTIVE:

➡ to understand the importance of converting positions into interests when resolving workplace conflict.

MATERIALS NEEDED: A copy of the case study on the following page for all participants

PROCEDURE:

Explain the difference between *positions* (what each party wants; the stated needs or demands) versus *interests* (the underlying reasons for what is wanted). Then engage participants in a discussion about the case with the questions below.

DEBRIEFING:

1 What are Tanya's positions and interests? What are Nancy's?
2 Does Tanya have valid concerns? Does Nancy?
3 How are Tanya's complaints affecting her nursing colleagues and others?
4 Do the needs of Olympian Hospital trump Tanya's individual needs in this case? Why or why not?
5 Are there ways for Nancy to address some, if not all, of Tanya's concerns while meeting the needs of the hospital?
6 What does this case teach us about handling conflict on the basis of mutual interests rather than positions?

CASE STUDY: NOT MY JOB

Tanya Harping, RN, began working at Olympian Hospital about four months ago and ever since, she has made it clear to anyone who will listen that she feels she is being inappropriately utilized. Tanya points out that on various occasions she has been asked to clean floors, do paperwork, and handle other tasks that non-clinical staff should handle. She also notes that administrators and the medical staff treat her like a second-class citizen, even referring to her a member of the "support staff," which annoys her greatly.

Some nurses are glad that Tanya is speaking up about their rights, while others don't want to work with her because they are tired of her complaints. The nursing supervisor, Nancy Carrington, RN, is at her wits end; sure, she asked Tanya to do some "non-nursing" activities, but the unit is short-staffed, everyone is busy, and she wants everyone to function like a team.

Nancy told Tanya that she would like nothing more than to hire more personnel, but the hospital has faced severe budgetary cutbacks and there is a hiring freeze at the current time. She criticized Tanya for not acting like a team player and said that she has "had it" with Tanya's attitude. Feeling that she was verbally slapped by this admonishment, Tanya is even more vocal about her concerns and has threatened to take the issue to the hospital administrator.

Despite the aggravation of working with Tanya, Nancy doesn't want her to resign. If she does, the unit would be even more short-handed than it is now and it would put even greater stress on the other nurses.

Moonlight in your eyes

TYPE: Case study

ESTIMATED TRAINING TIME: 30 minutes

THEMES: Conflict management, negotiation, difficult colleagues

OBJECTIVE:

➡ to gain experience dealing with conflicts involving a clash between individual and organizational needs.

MATERIALS NEEDED: A copy of the case study on the following page for all participants

PROCEDURE:

Ask the group for examples of instances in which a health care professional's personal needs are in conflict with those of their health care organization. Note that many such examples relate to the use of time and the life/work balance in people's lives. Then present the case study to participants.

DEBRIEFING:

1 Was Ms. May justified in thinking that Dr. Madison's quality of care could suffer from over-extending himself?
2 Does Dr. Madison have a point that what he does on his own time is his own concern? Why or why not?
3 What, if any, are their mutual interests?
4 What strategies would you recommend for resolving this conflict?

CASE STUDY: MOONLIGHT IN YOUR EYES

Dr. David Madison is a family physician who practices at the Blue Moon Health Center. Because he has enormous personal debts and a growing family, he believes it is essential to moonlight as much as possible. In addition to his responsibility at Blue Moon, he works periodically at a long-term care facility, a rehabilitation hospital, and a small medical center approximately 35 miles away.

This morning, the clinic director, Maddie Mays, has asked Dr. Madison to cut back on his moonlighting because he seems tired all the time. She explained that she has seen him yawning in mid-sentence, wiping his eyes, and nearly falling asleep on frequent visits to the health center's break room. Although Ms. Mays couldn't point to any evidence that a patient's care had suffered as a result of Dr. Madison's weariness, she suggested that it would only be a matter of time until a preventable problem occurred.

Dr. Madison protested strongly, noting that the extra workload had not adversely affected his quality of care and that he had a better idea than Ms. Mays about what he was able to handle. "No one cares about my patients more than I do," he said angrily, resenting the director's implications. He pointed out that he moonlighted throughout his residency training as well, and that he has learned to function quite well on three to four hours of sleep. He also believes that what he does in his private time is none of Ms. Mays' business.

Ms. Mays believes that the health center's needs come first and is adamant that Dr. Madison substantially reduce or discontinue his moonlighting if he is to continue his employment at Blue Moon. Dr. Madison has decided to have another discussion with Ms. Mays to try to resolve the situation amicably. He believes that he must keep working all these jobs; most of his income comes from the Blue Moon Health Center, but it is not enough to pay his mounting bills.

A disheartening situation

TYPE: Case study

ESTIMATED TRAINING TIME: 30 minutes

THEMES: Conflict management, negotiation, organizational change

OBJECTIVES:
➡ to identify issues in a conflict that involve the use of organizational resources;
➡ to show the importance of identifying both short-term and long-term needs.

MATERIALS NEEDED: A copy of the case study on the following page for all participants

PROCEDURE:
Beginning with a discussion about the rapid changes in medical technologies, divide the group into small groups, distribute the case study, and ask each group to discuss the issues involved in this conflict and how they believe it should be handled. Announce that the group will have 15 minutes to discuss the case and develop recommendations. After 15 minutes, bring everyone together for an all-group discussion.

DEBRIEFING:
1 What issues must Drs. Ventricle and Orta sort out as they try to resolve this conflict?
2 Does your group believe that the practice should purchase the new camera? Why or why not? Were other options discussed, such as renting or leasing a camera or buying a pre-owned, refurbished one?
3 Was it suggested that additional information be obtained before a decision could be made? If so, what type of information would be necessary? Why?
4 What are the practice's short-term needs? What are the long-term needs?
5 What can Dr. Orta do or say that will help Dr. Ventricle avoid seeing the purchase of the new echo as needless risk-taking?
6 Did your group address the issue of obsolescence; i.e. replacing a camera that is still working? How did your group believe that differences regarding new expenditures could be reconciled?

CASE STUDY: A DISHEARTENING SITUATION

Heartville Cardiology Associates (HCA) is a cardiology/thoracic surgery group practice with 10 physicians. HCA was established five years ago when six cardiologists and thoracic surgeons who worked together at a local multi-specialty group practice decided to split off and create their own group. Since that time, four more physicians have been added.

One of the group members is Dr. Lefty Ventricle, a senior partner and one of the founding members of the group. Dr. Ventricle, who currently serves as the group's president, is about five years from retirement and is extremely protective of the practice's assets. Another member of the group, Dr. A. Orta, joined the group two years ago straight from residency training. She is extremely excited about being part of the group, and wants to play a major role in the practice's growth and development.

During recent months, a major conflict has developed between Drs. Ventricle and Orta. Specifically, Dr. Orta wants to see the group take advantage of the latest technologies and upgrade its equipment. Specifically, she and another doctor want to purchase a new state-of-the-art echocardiogram that offers vastly improved imaging. It would cost $250 000. Dr. Ventricle opposes this because the practice already has an echocardiogram that was acquired from the old multi-specialty group practice. Since it was paid for several years ago and works quite well, Dr. Ventricle believes there's no need to replace it, even though the old echo doesn't have the capacity or the features of the new one. Other members of the group are neutral on this issue and want to see what Drs. Ventricle and Orta work out.

While Dr. Ventricle has noted that the practice's revenues have decreased during the past year and that it's not the right time to buy, Dr. Orta believes that the new echo will be an investment in the future, help to ensure that the practice is up-to-date, and increase revenues over the next 10 years. Dr. Ventricle wonders if he is the only one in the practice who cares about the practice's financial viability. He does not see why it is necessary to make such a major purchase when the current echo is still in good shape. It worries Dr. Ventricle to leave the practice in the hands of Dr. Orta and others who seem not to care about spending. Dr. Orta sees Dr. Ventricle as too fiscally conservative, seeing the issue as a matter of quality and keeping up with the times.

Staff members deal
with hurt feelings
and resentments
as they heal from
conflict

Letting bygones be bygones

TYPE: Case study

ESTIMATED TRAINING TIME: 30 minutes

THEMES: Conflict management, difficult colleagues, emotional intelligence

OBJECTIVE:

➡ to recognize the need for healing in the aftermath of a conflict.

MATERIALS NEEDED: A copy of the case on the next page for all participants

PROCEDURE:

After distributing copies of the case study, point out that people often think a conflict is over after an issue is resolved, but that hurt feelings and resentments may linger for a long time to come. Ask the group to develop recommendations on how the characters in this case study should facilitate their post-conflict healing.

DEBRIEFING:

1   After Jackie Daniels, RN, was selected as the new head of nursing, Johnny Redd and Sally Smirnoff had no more reason to bicker. So why did the tensions continue?
2   What are the undercurrents in the relationship between Johnny and Sally?
3   Should Sally have confronted Johnny about the rumor? Why or why not? How could she have avoided Johnny's defensiveness?
4   What could Johnny and/or Sally do to rebuild their working relationship and, possibly, their friendship?
5   What role can Jackie Daniels play in the healing process?

CASE STUDY: LETTING BYGONES BE BYGONES

When Jackie Daniels, RN, was hired as the new head of the nursing department at Grey Goose Hospital, it seemed that all of the internal turmoil in the department would finally abate. After serving in management at a medical center in another State for the previous 20 years, Ms. Daniels decided to apply for this position so that she could live closer to her ailing sister. Hospital administration had a welcoming reception for Ms. Daniels when she arrived, and toasted her as "the most qualified person for this important job" and "the best choice we could have made."

During the previous six months, after the former nursing director, Kendy Jackson, RN, had announced her retirement, several of the nurses began to speculate who the new head of nursing would be. Most members of the nursing staff assumed that Sally Smirnoff, RN, MSN, would be the odds-on choice, but Johnny Redd, RN, made it known that he was interested in the position as well.

Even before Johnny formally applied for the job, he began a department-wide campaign to gain support from his colleagues. In his discussions, he often noted that Sally had not worked at Grey Goose Hospital as long as he had (6 years, compared with his 14 years), and suggested that Sally's personal problems (a nasty divorce and child custody battle that made the local newspapers) would impede her ability to manage the department effectively. He told one of his colleagues that he'd heard that Sally recently had gotten "plastered" in a local bar, to the point that she had to be assisted home. "Is this the type of person we want in this position?" he asked.

Several of Sally's friends told her about Johnny's comments. She confronted him privately, telling him that she had gone through quite a lot from her abusive ex-husband and that it was very painful to be "abused" by a colleague as well. She vociferously denied that she was ever in the bar that Johnny mentioned, much less that she had too much to drink. "I am home every night with my children," she noted. "They need me now more than ever."

Johnny said that he had heard the rumors about Sally, but denied spreading them himself. He said he'd never say such a thing because it would backfire on him as he tried to build support for his candidacy. "What a liar," Sally said. "I don't know what's happened to you over the last few months, but you've become a selfish backstabber. I hope you can live with yourself."

"I have no problem sleeping at night, Sally," Johnny responded. "I just hope the things I've heard about you are not true."

* * *

It didn't take long for Jackie Daniels to detect the undercurrent of tension when she arrived. She set up private meetings with each member of her staff to exchange information about their expectations, and during these talks she learned quite a bit about the lingering resentments – not just between Sally and Johnny, but also among several nurses who aligned themselves with one or the other. Other nurses were hopeful that the tensions would die down after Jackie had a chance to demonstrate her leadership and management skills.

* * *

"I just don't believe what's happened," Sally said to her friend, Glenna Livet, LPN, after their shifts were over. "The last few months have been horrible. On top of my personal problems, I keep thinking of the horrible things that Johnny Redd said about me, and now they've selected someone from another State to be the new Director of Nursing. I've worked so hard here; I can't believe they went 'outside' to fill the position."

"Yes, but you do have to admit that Jackie knows what she's doing," Glenna said. "It's kind of good to have some fresh perspectives. Say, are you and Johnny getting along any better these days?"

"We barely talk," Sally replied. "I can't believe he used to be one of the people I felt closest to here. Now it's hard to know what to believe."

Just then, Johnny approached. After exchanging hellos, Sally tried to force a smile. "Hey Johnny, I've been meaning to ask you. How do you like our new director?"

"Well, I hate to admit it, but she's not bad. I would have been better, of course!"

Sally laughed. "Actually, I think this is going to work out very well. In fact, Jackie just asked me to head our quality improvement committee, and I'm very excited about it."

"Really? I happen to know a lot about quality improvement myself," Johnny said. "Add my name to your committee roster, okay?"

Sally pretended like she didn't hear his comment. Could she trust him? Would he try to undermine her from within her own committee? Was this a ploy?

The Doctor-in-the-Brochure

TYPE: Case study

ESTIMATED TRAINING TIME: 60 minutes

THEMES: Conflict management, negotiation

OBJECTIVES:

➡ to show the dynamics and issues involved in intra-specialty conflict;

➡ to explore the role and evolution of modern day family medicine.

MATERIALS NEEDED: Copies of the case study and discussion sheet for all participants; table-top flip charts and markers are desirable for each table, but not required.

PROCEDURE:

Divide participants into groups of five to seven persons each and ask them to read the case study and try to come to consensus on questions listed on the Discussion Sheet. Tell the groups they will have 35 minutes to try to reach agreement on as many questions as they can.

DEBRIEFING:

After the small-group discussions, point out that the purpose of this exercise was not just to air their views about the questions on the Discussion Sheet, but also to see how the group handled any conflicts that arose among group participants. Then ask:

1 What areas did members of your group agree most strongly about? In what areas did you disagree?

2 How did your group handle dissension? Were minority opinions respected? Did those who spoke the loudest or the longest have greater influence on the group's decision making than those with more moderate views?

3 Did group members actively listen to one another? Were follow-up questions asked to clarify other group members' views?

4 Assuming that there were disagreements within your group, were they handled effectively? What improvements would you suggest?

Author's note: While many family physicians have tailored the scope of their practices to fit personal preferences, I personally know that the most important features of the Doctor-in-the-Brochure still exist. Thanks to my doctor and model for the D-I-B, Lawrence Houston, MD, of Overland Park, Kansas! – EJB

CASE STUDY: THE DOCTOR-IN-THE-BROCHURE

After cleaning out files at your family medicine residency program, you found an old brochure entitled, "The New Specialty of Family Practice" that was written back in the early 1970s, shortly after being designated as a specialty in 1969. You couldn't wait to share portions of the old brochure at the next faculty meeting.

You opened the faculty meeting by starting with the brochure's title. Several faculty members laughed knowingly, noting that the specialty is now referred to as family medicine. You continued reading:

> "Like the general practitioners of yesteryear, the family physician is a specialist that provides continuing, comprehensive care throughout the patient's lifetime – from cradle to grave – and treats between 80% and 95% of the problems, complaints, and conditions for which a patient sees a doctor."

You read several other portions of the brochure, which stated that the family physician treats all members of the family "in breadth and in depth," knows the complete family history (which contributes to quality care), and is known for excellent listening skills and providing "care with caring." It also says:

> "The family physician is the only specialist that still provides house calls."

You suggested that the rest of the meeting should be devoted to a discussion of how family medicine has evolved – and how it should continue to evolve – since that may affect the development of curricula for tomorrow's family medicine specialist.

"Does the 'Doctor-in-the-Brochure' still exist?" you asked. "Should we train our residents to be that doctor, or should we train our residents in the way they intend to practice in accordance with our changing times and each doctor's practice preferences?"

DISCUSSION QUESTIONS

1 In what ways is today's family medicine specialist still like the "Doctor-in-the-Brochure" (D-I-B)? What *hasn't* changed – at least by much?
2 What changes in the health care industry or in society have enabled family physicians to make more choices today about their scope of practice than the general practitioners of yesteryear were able to do?
3 How have these changes benefited today's family medicine specialist? Their patients?

4 Have any of the changes gone too far? Are there parts of the D-I-B that should be brought back?

5 In what ways has the evolution from the D-I-B of the 1970s to today's family physician helped or hindered relationships with other specialties? With patients?

6 Should residents continue to be trained in both hospital and ambulatory settings? Or should those that plan to assign their patients to a "hospitalist" be trained in ambulatory settings only?

7 In what ways do family physicians provide continuing and comprehensive care to their patients today – regardless of their scope of practice?

8 Is cradle-to-grave care a thing of the past? Or should this type of care be revisited?

Six cases that
explore gender
conflicts in health
care settings

Gender conflicts

TYPE: Case studies

ESTIMATED TRAINING TIME: 30 minutes

THEMES: Conflict management, negotiation, difficult colleagues

OBJECTIVES:

➡ to understand the issues and sensitivities involved in gender-related conflicts;

➡ to identify ways of resolving gender conflicts while maintaining and perhaps improving working relationships.

MATERIALS NEEDED: A copy of two selected cases for all participants

PROCEDURE:

Distribute two selected cases from the following pages and discuss the cases in all-group or small-group discussions. Your choices are:

➡ **What is fair?** – Female physicians in a large primary care group practice seek time off to be with their young children, to the dismay of their male counterparts.

➡ **The joker is wild** – A nurse complains to the practice manager about offensive jokes being told by a physician and physician assistant.

➡ **Building bonds** – Nurses and administrative staff in a rural practice experience tensions as a result of working with a female physician for the first time.

➡ **Medicine woman** – A 73-year-old male patient wants to be fit into the schedule for an office visit, but does not want to be treated by a female physician.

➡ **Mars and Venus** – Female nurses seem to treat a female physician differently than male physicians – and the male physicians think that's acceptable.

➡ **Gender bias**[1] – Male physicians in a family medicine residency complain that they are not being adequately trained in treating female patients.

Either in small groups or the group as a whole, ask participants to address the questions following each case, as well as any other questions that occur to them.

---

1   A special thanks to Susan Zeltzer, MD, a faculty member of Providence Family Medicine Residency in Southfield, Michigan, for developing the scenario in Gender Bias.

CASE STUDY: WHAT IS FAIR?

The 15 partners of a large primary group practice are about to meet to discuss a major conflict. Of the five female partners, two have small children and one is pregnant; these three physicians would like to work fewer hours to spend time with family while their children are growing up. The other two female physicians support their colleagues' request even though they wish to continue working full-time.

The 10 male physicians are very upset about this request; they believe that all partners should be working more, not less, in order to boost productivity and practice revenues.

"We have kids too, but we're not asking for time off – why should you?" the male doctors ask.

Revenues are particularly essential because of plans for a much-needed practice renovation. What advice would you give this group?

DISCUSSION QUESTIONS

1 What are the key issues involved in this conflict? To what extent are gender issues involved?
2 Does the reason that the female physicians are seeking time off actually matter in this dispute? Why or why not?
3 What strategies would help to resolve this conflict?
4 What creative solutions would you recommend?

CASE STUDY: THE JOKER IS WILD

As the practice manager in your community health center, a nurse recently complained to you about a physician and physician assistant who often tell off-color jokes, many of which are about women. They have been very careful to tell these jokes in small groups, not in the presence of patients, but the nurse is offended by their jokes nonetheless. Some jokes have sexual overtones, and some are "dumb-blonde" jokes.

In the past, when you have asked the physician and physician assistant to refrain from this behavior, they called you hypocritical because they've seen you laugh at some of their jokes before. (You actually find the two of them quite amusing.)

You would like to maintain good working relationships and a good atmosphere – this physician and physician assistant are excellent clinicians and would be hard to replace – and you'd prefer not to be in a policing role. As a practice leader, what should you do?

DISCUSSION QUESTIONS

1   What are the differences in perspectives between the parties involved in this conflict?
2   Since patients have not heard these jokes, should the practice manager be concerned about the nurse's complaints? Why or why not?
3   Are there any points in favor of the physician and physician assistant?
4   What are the likely outcomes if the practice manager does not address this issue?
5   How can the practice manager address this issue without taking on the role of "office police"?

CASE STUDY: BUILDING BONDS

A recent residency graduate, Belinda Blender, DO, has just entered practice in a rural community to replace a physician who retired. The previous physician, who had established the practice 40 years ago, was reminiscent of the television character, Marcus Welby, MD – a grandfatherly type who was beloved throughout the community. When he retired, nurses and administrative staff were nervous about the changing dynamics; in addition to being sad that they had lost the practice's patriarch, they had never worked with a female physician before!

Dr. Blender felt the strain immediately. The more it seemed that people acted awkwardly around her – with some even trying to keep their distance – the more Dr. Blender felt that she was "out of the loop." Although she had an office next to the other physicians on the second floor, she moved her desk near the nursing station on the first floor, not far from the administrative offices. She said this move was so that she could build bonds with the women who worked in the practice as well as to be in the center of activity.

Nurses have complained to the office manager that they resent the doctor being in their area. They perceive this as a way to keep tabs on their every move or, as one nurse put it, "to spy on us." Several administrative staff members said that they can't figure out why Dr. Blender wouldn't keep her office in proximity to the other doctors and feel suspicious of her move. What should Dr. Blender do?

DISCUSSION QUESTIONS

1 What issues are involved in this conflict, aside from gender?
2 Should efforts be made to address this conflict individually, or as a group? Explain your response.
3 How should this conflict be handled?
4 Should Dr. Blender move back to her office on the second floor rather than work near the nursing station? Explain your response.
5 What else can Dr. Blender do to build better relationships with nurses and administrative staff members?

CASE STUDY: MEDICINE WOMAN

A relatively new patient, a 73-year-old male with a long list of health problems, has asked to be fit into the schedule for an office visit because of flu-like symptoms, which he suspects is West Nile Virus. No one else can fit this patient in except Michelle Quinn, DO. When the receptionist told this patient which doctor would be able to see him, she added, "You will really like her; she's great!" Hearing the word "she," the patient expressed concern about being seen by a female physician.

The receptionist asked Dr. Quinn if she would speak to the patient to assuage his concerns, and she agreed, seeing this as a "teachable moment." What should Dr. Quinn do or say to put this patient at ease?

DISCUSSION QUESTIONS

1   If you are Dr. Quinn, how will you begin this conversation with the patient?
2   What questions will you ask in order to find out what is behind the patient's concerns?
3   What types of things might the patient hesitate to say to your face?
4   How can you put the patient at ease about seeing you?
5   How do you think this situation might be different if the patient was female and the doctor was male? Would this still be a teachable moment?

CASE STUDY: MARS AND VENUS

As a female physician, you have noticed a huge difference in how nurses treat you in comparison to how they treat your male counterparts. When male physicians in your practice seemed stressed, staff members act very supportively. But when you appear stressed, they make every effort to avoid you. What's more, the nurses frequently refer to you by your first name – not in front of patients, though – even though they always refer to the male physicians as "Doctor." When you mentioned this to one of the nurses, she said that they meant no disrespect; it was because the male doctors are so much older than you.

At today's all-staff meeting, you voiced your concerns about being treated differently than the males in the office. One of your male colleagues began to laugh. "The staff is behaving quite normally," he said. "I'll bet you even treat your female and male patients somewhat differently, don't you?" he asked.

DISCUSSION QUESTIONS

1 Should you have brought up this concern in an all-staff meeting? Why or why not?
2 How should you respond to the comment that staff was behaving normally?
3 To what extent was the issue about gender? About age?
4 What, if anything, should the female physician say to staff members that she perceives are avoiding her? Should she address gender specifically?
5 Physical differences and clinical needs aside, do physicians tend to treat male and female *patients* differently? If so, how?

CASE STUDY: GENDER BIAS

A family medicine residency has two teaching offices: one in a large metropolitan area and the other in a small rural community. The rural office, which was established by three female faculty physicians, frequently has more female residents than male residents. Over the years, female patients in the rural office have tended to see a female physician for routine physical examinations and pelvic exams, even if their primary provider in the office is a male. Because the male residents have very few women on their schedules for preventive medicine examinations, they feel that they are being inadequately trained to do them.

Although the faculty recognizes the problem, they are unsure how to change a pattern that has existed for more than 20 years. The medical director of the rural office tried to investigate, but isn't certain whether female patients have been insisting on seeing a woman for routine examinations or whether the receptionist who is scheduling the appointments is biased toward scheduling in this manner. The residency's metropolitan teaching office has never experienced this problem.

DISCUSSION QUESTIONS

1   If the problem is due to female patients requesting female physicians, do the faculty physicians violate any rights of these patients by trying to steer them to see the male residents?

2   Do the educational needs of the resident take preference over the requests of patients in certain circumstances?

3   If the problem is due to bias by the receptionist who schedules the appointments, what can the medical director and faculty do?

4   What phrases would a phone receptionist use to convince a female patient to see a male resident for her physical?

5   How would the faculty change a long-standing "culture" of women-treating-women that seems to exist within the office as well as with their patient population?

6   Why did this bias develop in the rural office? What practices could have been put in place to prevent such a bias from developing?

Training Tool #20

A dose of reality

TYPE: Role play – five characters

ESTIMATED TRAINING TIME: 90 minutes

THEMES: Conflict management, negotiation

OBJECTIVE:

➥ explore ways to deal with a multi-party conflict involving parents, school administration, and school nurses – all of whom have a child's best interests at heart.

MATERIALS NEEDED: A copy of the General Instructions for all participants, and a copy of individual instructions for the five characters in each group

PROCEDURE:

Divide participants into groups of five. Distribute the General Instructions to everyone, and give instructions for a different role to each person in the small groups. Participants will know what role they will play by the instruction sheet they receive.

After allowing about 5–10 minutes for review of the material, instruct each group to role play this case for 45 minutes and try to come up with a solution that is acceptable to all parties (if possible) and that takes into account the child's best interests.

DEBRIEFING:

1 How effectively did your group handle this conflict? Did you achieve a mutual-gains solution? What solution did your group accept?

2 What strategies were most helpful in resolving this situation? If your group reached an impasse, what contributed to that?

3 What actions were taken to neutralize Edith's and Archie's emotional outbursts? Were they successful?

4 If this case occurred in real life, what could the school nurse administrator and/or the school nurse do to handle this conflict more successfully?

ROLE PLAY: A DOSE OF REALITY
GENERAL INSTRUCTIONS

Players
- Mr. Archie Bonkers, father of Billy Bonkers
- Mrs. Edith Bonkers, mother of Billy Bonkers
- Frieda Fine, RN, school nurse at Happyville Elementary School
- Mary Mediator, RN, school nurse administrator for Great Independent School District
- Sara Schoolhead, principal of Happyville Elementary School

Billy Bonkers is a precocious six-year old boy who has been absent from school a great deal this year due to a variety of illnesses (infections, asthma, tonsillitis, flu, colds, etc.) Not long ago, Billy's mother, Edith Bonkers, came to Happyville Elementary School to visit with the school nurse, Frieda Fine, RN. During this visit, she handed Mrs. Fine a bottle of medications that she said would help to build up Billy's immune system. "Please be sure that Billy takes one of these pills before lunch every day," she asked.

Mrs. Fine became suspicious the minute she saw the container. It was not an over-the-counter (OTC) medication, and the label said, "Nogales, Mexico." Mrs. Fine politely explained that it was contrary to school policy to administer medications that are brought in from another country. She pointed out that they are only allowed to administer OTC medications or those that are prescribed by the child's physician.

Mrs. Bonkers became very angry and called her husband, Archie. Upon getting the call from his wife, Mr. Bonkers became so upset that he left work and drove to the school. Mrs. Fine couldn't seem to convince the Bonkers that she had valid reasons for not agreeing to give Billy the pills. Mr. Bonkers pounded his fist on the table, saying that the school was interfering with his parental rights to care for his child as he sees fit. Mrs. Bonkers yelled at Mrs. Fine and called her names. Then Mrs. Bonkers started crying.

Mrs. Fine calmly told the Bonkers that she would contact the school nurse administrator for the Great Independent School District (Mary Mediator, RN) to identify ways to deal with this issue. Ms. Mediator suggested that they set up a meeting with the Bonkers and ask the school principal, Sara Schoolhead, to join the group as well.

That meeting is about to begin.

ROLE PLAY: A DOSE OF REALITY
CONFIDENTIAL INSTRUCTIONS

Mr. Archie Bonkers [Billy Bonker's father]

You have a short fuse anyway (you've been treated for an anger control problem in the past), but the people at Happyville Elementary School are REALLY pressing your hot buttons. The reason you're so upset is that you think it's terrible that the school won't respect the wishes of parents regarding the care of their own child. The school allows one of Billy's friends to maintain his vegetarian diet at the school – even though you consider that wrong since the kid will probably get anemic. Why does the school trust other parents' judgment but not yours?

It breaks your heart that Billy gets sick so much, and even though you yell too much at home, you consider yourself a good dad. It has cost you a fortune to take Billy to several doctors; after all, your family is underinsured. No one seemed able to figure out Billy's problem until you and Edith took Billy to an alternative medicine clinic in Nogales, Mexico. The doctor there was quite sure that Billy had an immune deficiency – one that could be cured with a "miracle drug" that was available only through that clinic. It was quite expensive (a six-month supply was $4000), but you borrowed the money to pay for it.

You've noticed major improvements in Billy's health during the 30 days since he's been taking the drug. He hasn't missed one day of school since! Your wife, Edith, had been giving Billy his pill every day when Billy came home for lunch, but Edith is starting a new job next week to help pay off this new debt. The pill is supposed to be taken with meals, so it's imperative that Billy gets his mid-day pill right before lunch. Giving Billy his pills in the morning and evening are not a problem since you and your wife are with him then.

At today's meeting, you will try to get the school to understand what your family has been going through, and that you and Edith have Billy's best interests at heart. You are quite resistant to taking Billy off this drug as nothing else has seemed to work. You want the school to make an exception to their policy and give Billy his medication while you and Edith are at work. If you feel that you're not being listened to, you plan to threaten a lawsuit.

Note: Display some rage during the early part of this meeting and see what the others do to calm you down. If the strategies they use would work in real life, you can then act more rationally.

ROLE PLAY: A DOSE OF REALITY
CONFIDENTIAL INSTRUCTIONS

Mrs. Edith Bonkers [Billy Bonker's mother]

It makes you mad that your husband can be such a hothead, but this time you don't blame him one bit!

The reason you're so upset is that you consider yourself to be an excellent mother. You love your son Billy more than anything and would never do anything to hurt him. You have taken Billy to many doctors, but none of them could figure out why he gets sick all the time. The only doctor who made any sense at all to you and your husband, Archie, is a doctor from Nogales, Mexico, who was recommended to you by some advocates of alternative medicine that you met at a PTA meeting.

The doctor in Nogales said that Billy's immune system was quite weak and that he had a "miracle drug" that would help him. He assured you that the drug was extremely safe, and pointed out that it is only available at his clinic. (It has not been FDA approved.) You ordered a six-month supply; it was extremely expensive, but you and Archie borrowed $4000 to pay for it.

Billy has been taking this drug for 30 days and has not had one symptom since. Billy has had no side effects from the drug. During this time, you've been giving Billy his pill when he came home for lunch. Giving Billy his morning and evening pills is no problem since you and your husband are with him then, but you don't want him to miss his mid-day pill, which you've been told must be taken with lunch. However, next week you're starting a new job (to help pay the debt of this medication!) and you can't take time off from work. You want the school to respect your wishes and give your son the medication as you have instructed. Although they haven't said it directly, you don't like it that school nurses and officials seem to be accusing you of being a bad parent.

Note: You are very emotional and defensive — especially at the beginning of this meeting. See what the other parties do to try to neutralize your emotions. If their strategies would work in real life, you can then act more rationally.

ROLE PLAY: A DOSE OF REALITY
CONFIDENTIAL INSTRUCTIONS

Frieda Fine, RN [School Nurse at Happyville Elementary School]
You have been a school nurse at Happyville Elementary School for 20 years, and you take great pride in "doing things by the book." You are highly respected by teachers as well as administration. Your personal motto is "Put children first."

When Mrs. Bonkers handed you the bottle of pills that she wanted you to administer to Billy at lunchtime everyday, you were not surprised that the label said, "Nogales, Mexico." Several other parents have frequented the same alternative medicine clinic, and you have faced this problem before. The other parents have listened to reason about school policy, which strictly forbids the administration of any drug that is obtained in another country. Unlike the other parents, Mr. and Mrs. Bonkers don't seem to listen.

While you take great pride in your ability to deal with parents effectively, the Bonkers were so emotional at your previous meeting with them that you called your school nurse administrator, Mary Mediator, RN, for help and advice. You realize that you've gotten emotionally involved in this case. You don't trust the medication that Billy has been given and are deeply concerned about possible long-term effects on Billy's health. On a personal level, you are also upset with the Bonkers because they have been resisting your authority and personal judgment.

You also wonder whether the principal (Sara Schoolhead) is truly supportive of you. Shortly before today's meeting, you had a major falling out with her. At a meeting with Sara, you said, "I can't give Billy the pills – it's not only against our school policy, it's against the law!" Sara replied, "Well, *I'm* the principal and *I* give you permission. Let *me* worry about the law." You stormed out of Sara's office, and haven't seen her again until today.

ROLE PLAY: A DOSE OF REALITY
CONFIDENTIAL INSTRUCTIONS

Sara Schoolhead [Principal of Happyville Elementary School]

As the principal of Happyville Elementary School, you've been making a lot of efforts during recent years to improve relationships with parents. You've had to deal with a lot of irate parents lately, so keeping things on an even keel has been quite a chore.

You've been dealing with two lawsuits from other parents lately, and you'd do almost anything to avoid another one. Generally, you believe that all school policies should be followed, and that the principal should stand by the judgment of the school nurse. On the other hand, if Frieda wasn't so hardheaded about this issue, there would be no more problem – no threat of another lawsuit!

Personally, you don't see why Frieda is so adamant, especially since the pills that the Bonkers are giving Billy have no proven harm. (You've been wondering, what's the big deal about giving someone an herbal remedy? People get herbs from health food stores all the time!) Unfortunately, you had a falling out with Frieda shortly before today's meeting. A day or so ago, Frieda came into your office and said, "I can't give Billy the pills – it's not only against our school policy, it's against the law!" In the interest of putting this issue to rest, you replied, "Well, *I'm* the principal and *I* give you permission. Let *me* worry about the law." Frieda stormed out of your office.

You have also wondered to yourself whether Frieda could have done more to resolve this problem quietly with the Bonkers without having to drag you into it. You don't know Mary Mediator, the school nurse administrator, very well, but you have felt a little competitive with her in the past. If you had your way, you'd like to have those who attend today's meeting see *you* as the key problem-solver, not her.

ROLE PLAY: A DOSE OF REALITY
CONFIDENTIAL INSTRUCTIONS

Mary Mediator, RN [School Nurse Administrator for the Great Independent School District]

You know you're walking into a bad situation – after all, Frieda Fine is one of your most effective staff members when it comes to dealing with irate parents. Since Frieda had difficulty dealing with them at a previous meeting, you know you'll have your hands full!

So far, you've only talked to Frieda about this situation, and you haven't talked to Mr. or Mrs. Bonkers yet. You're anxious to hear more about their perspectives at today's meeting, but so far you agree with Frieda in this situation. You feel that she's absolutely right: giving the unauthorized drug to Billy will violate school policy. On the other hand, you want to demonstrate to the parents that you are respectful of their role.

You haven't had a chance to tell Frieda yet, but you have done some research on the drug that Billy is being given prior to this meeting. The drug is mostly herbal, and the components seem to be nontoxic when given in limited dosages. However, the effects on children have not been sufficiently tested. You are concerned about the long-term effects, even though you do have anecdotal evidence from other parents whose children have taken similar medications for long periods without serious side effects. (Whether you mention any or all of this at the meeting is up to you.)

You are also aware of a rift between Frieda Fine and Sara Schoolhead. As Frieda reported to you, she recently went into Sara's office and said, "I can't give Billy the pills – it's not only against our school policy, it's against the law!" Sara replied, "Well, *I'm* the principal and *I* give you permission. Let *me* worry about the law." Frieda said that she stormed out of Sara's office. You are concerned that if this rift surfaces at the meeting, the school won't appear to have a unified front.

A dispute between
two physicians
concerning the call
schedule

It's your call

TYPE: Role play – two physicians: Dr. Painhart and Dr. Goodly

ESTIMATED TRAINING TIME: 30 minutes

THEMES: Conflict management, negotiation, difficult colleagues

OBJECTIVES:

➡ to demonstrate how people's expectations of one another and perceptions of
unfairness can contribute to workplace conflict;

➡ to show how interpersonal conflicts involving fairness issues can be successfully
resolved.

MATERIALS NEEDED: Copies of the two roles for each dyad

PROCEDURE:

Ask participants to identify a partner. If there are an uneven number of participants, have
the extra person serve as observer. Distribute the confidential instructions for the roles
of Drs. Painhart and Goodly so that each person in the dyad is playing an opposing role.
Announce that the group will have 15 minutes to conduct the role play.

DEBRIEFING:

1   What were the issues in this case? What were the differences between Dr. Painhart's
needs and interests and those of Dr. Goodly?

2   Was Dr. Painhart unreasonable in expecting Dr. Goodly to take even more call after six
months? Why or why not?

3   Did it matter that the extra call would be so that Dr. Painhart could train for a triathlon?
Was it more acceptable when Dr. Painhart needed time away from call for marriage
counseling? In other words, do reasons matter?

4   Who set the tone in the conversation about this problem? What was the effect of starting
the discussion in that way?

5   What process did you use to resolve the conflict? In retrospect, what would you do
differently?

6   Was the conflict resolved successfully? If so, how? How was the issue of fairness
handled, from the perspectives of both parties? Did you address the issue of immediate
versus long-term reciprocity?

ROLE PLAY: IT'S YOUR CALL
CONFIDENTIAL INSTRUCTIONS

Dr. Painhart

You are Dr. Painhart, a family physician who practices at Gladtown Family Medicine with your partner (another family physician), Dr. Goodly. You and Dr. Goodly have been in practice together for one year. You met at your residency program and have very similar practice styles. The patient load is extremely high; after all, you are the only family physicians in Gladtown, a small town with 5000 people and a drawing area of several thousand more. Your spouses are close friends.

Because you've had some major personal problems, you've asked Dr. Goodly to take call for you on many different occasions during the past six months. In previous months, you were concerned that your marriage was on the rocks; this was a devastating possibility, as you and your spouse were childhood sweethearts. While your marriage was in trouble, you needed numerous evenings off, not only to spend more time with your spouse, but also for all of the marriage counseling sessions that you and your spouse attended.

Now that your marriage issues have been resolved, you still plan to ask Dr. Goodly to take call for you several more times during the next two months. That's because you have been training for an upcoming triathlon. You feel confident about your cycling and running abilities, but you need a great deal more practice in the swimming component, particularly to build your endurance in frigid waters. The only lake in Gladtown has been polluted from industrial waste, so you plan to drive three evenings each week to Pleasantville Lake, which is 45 miles away. Because the lake is near a residential area and is well lit, you can swim there at night.

To date, Dr. Goodly hasn't seemed to mind taking call for you, but seems to be acting a little testy lately. Dr. Goodly has just walked into your office to speak with you. You have several reasons for asking Dr. Goodly to handle extra call during the next two months. First, you plan to be partners with Dr. Goodly for the rest of your career, and you know that you'll be able to more than compensate for this great favor in the months and years to come. Why do things have to even out every month? Second, completing the triathlon has been your lifelong dream, and you'd like to achieve this goal now while you still have the strength to get through the race. You have a family history of rheumatoid arthritis and you've noticed that your morning stiffness is getting worse. You feel it's essential to do this triathlon now – while you still can.

ROLE PLAY: IT'S YOUR CALL
CONFIDENTIAL INSTRUCTIONS

Dr. Goodly

You are a family physician, Dr. Goodly, who practices at Gladtown Family Medicine with your partner (another family physician), Dr. Painhart. You and Dr. Painhart have been in practice together for one year. You met at your residency program, and have very similar practice styles. With Gladtown's population of 5000 and a surrounding area of several thousand more, your patient load is extremely high. Aside from the two of you, there are no other family physicians in town.

During the last six months, Dr. Painhart has been tremendously agitated, which you learned was due to marital problems. So that Dr. Painhart could spend more time at home and attend marriage counseling sessions during the evenings, you were very happy to help out by taking more than your share of call.

At first you were patient, but after six months, you began to feel that "enough is enough." Now that Dr. Painhart's marriage is back on track (a great relief, because you and your spouse are close friends of theirs), you are anxious to get back to an equitable call schedule. After all, doesn't Dr. Painhart realize that you have a life too?

You have just walked into Dr. Painhart's office to discuss the call schedule for the next few months. While simply sharing call equally would be a great relief, you would prefer that Dr. Painhart start taking more than half the call in the coming months in order to make up for all of your sacrifice on his behalf.

Surely Dr. Painhart would not have the nerve to ask you again to take more than your fair share of call anytime soon. If this were the case, you would feel that it would be strong evidence that your partner is taking advantage of you, and that would make you extremely angry. If an emergency arose, that would be one thing, but if Dr. Painhart asked you to take call for any other reason – like preparing for the "stupid" triathlon that is coming up – that would cause you to question the future of this partnership.

Dispute about filling
out procedures forms
on a timely basis

Training Tool #22

The paper chase

TYPE: Role play – administrator and physician

ESTIMATED TRAINING TIME: 30 minutes

THEMES: Conflict management, negotiation, difficult colleagues

OBJECTIVE:

➡ to demonstrate how conflicts stemming from time-management problems and differences in priorities can be successfully resolved.

MATERIALS NEEDED: Copies of the two roles for each dyad

PROCEDURE:

Ask all participants to identify a partner. If there are an uneven number of participants, have the extra person serve as observer. Distribute the confidential instructions for the administrator and physician so that each person in the dyads is playing an opposing role. Advise the group that they will have 15 minutes to complete the role play.

DEBRIEFING:

1   What is likely to happen if the conflict is not satisfactorily resolved?
2   Did the administrator offer warnings, threats, or ultimatums? If so, were other strategies applied first?
3   To what extent do the physician and administrator each have valid points?
4   Was the physician's workload addressed? How did the administrator handle the issue regarding the physician's relationship with billing clerks?
5   What processes and strategies were most effective for turning the dispute into a win-win situation?
6   Did your solutions meet the needs of the physician as well as the administrator?

ROLE PLAY: THE PAPER CHASE
CONFIDENTIAL INSTRUCTIONS

Administrator

You are the top administrator of an ambulatory care department in your academic medical center, and you've had a terrible month. For one thing, you had to terminate a physician who was not performing well and that caused a terrible morale problem among others who had to pick up the slack. Letting go of people is the hardest part of your job.

One of your biggest headaches lately has been an ongoing dispute with one of the physicians who sees patients in the health center and also serves as a faculty member. The main issue is that the physician has not seemed to be functioning as a team player. In particular, the physician does not complete the necessary procedure forms for his/her patients on a timely basis, which often delays the billing process. You have had several discussions with the physician about this issue, but they have not led to any major improvements.

You also are upset that the physician has been curt with the billing clerks who have returned forms to the physician when they were filled out incorrectly. You will speak to the physician now.

ROLE PLAY: THE PAPER CHASE
CONFIDENTIAL INSTRUCTIONS

Physician

You are a physician in the ambulatory care department at an academic medical center. You're getting tired of the top administrator coming to you week after week to complain that you are not completing the procedures forms for your health center patients in a timely manner. The truth is, you have been late with your forms, but there is no way around it. You are overwhelmed with work, and besides, your major responsibilities are to serve as a faculty member and clinician, not as a paper-pusher.

You also resent the administrator telling you how to treat other staff members. You've had some unpleasant encounters with the billing clerks, but you believe they were totally out of line to send forms back to you for correction over some very trivial points.

The administrator is now coming to your office for a talk.

Clinically speaking

TYPE: Role play – administrator and provider

ESTIMATED TRAINING TIME: 30 minutes

THEMES: Conflict management, difficult colleagues

OBJECTIVE:

➡ to demonstrate ways to resolve disputes involving professional boundaries and conflicting needs.

MATERIALS NEEDED: Copies of the two roles for each dyad

PROCEDURE:

Ask participants to identify a partner. If there are an uneven number of participants, have the extra person serve as observer. Distribute the confidential instructions for the administrator and provider so that each person in the dyads is playing an opposing role. Tell the group that they will have 15 minutes to conduct the role play.

DEBRIEFING:

1 What are the issues in this dispute?
2 Is it within the administrator's purview to suggest that the provider see more patients? Why or why not?
3 How did the provider feel about the administrator reviewing his/her charts? Would these feelings be justifiable?
4 To what extent, if any, is the provider's practice style an issue here? Should the provider be concerned with productivity? Why or why not? How can productivity be addressed without compromising the provider's desire to spend sufficient time with each patient?
5 How did the characters in each dyad reconcile their conflicting needs (i.e. the provider's practice style preferences versus the practice's needs for greater productivity)? What are the areas of common ground?
6 Were the solutions satisfactory to each party? What process and strategies were most effective?

ROLE PLAY: CLINICALLY SPEAKING
CONFIDENTIAL INSTRUCTIONS

Administrator

You are the administrator of Grand Community Health Center. Lately, you've been having a number of arguments with a new provider who feels that you've been getting too involved on the clinical side. Sure, you've been suggesting that the new provider see more patients in order to keep the numbers up, but you feel that it is your responsibility to point out the numbers. Your practice has only recently gotten out of the red, and you need to ensure the practice's viability. Besides, you've checked with other practices in the region, and their providers see about six more patients per day than your provider does.

You like to know exactly what has been going on in the practice and, although you haven't mentioned this before, you have been reviewing the provider's charts. You may not have done this if the provider didn't make you question his/her productivity level, but you wanted to see if there were other issues too. Even after reviewing the charts, you still can't figure out why more patients haven't been seen.

ROLE PLAY: CLINICALLY SPEAKING
CONFIDENTIAL INSTRUCTIONS

Provider

You are the new provider at Grand Community Health Center. You've been extremely upset with the administrator lately, who you feel has been getting much too involved in the clinical side of the practice. The administrator keeps telling you to increase your productivity, and to see at least six more patients per day.

You feel that you barely spend enough time with your patients as it is, and that if you see more patients it could adversely affect your ability to provide quality service and quality care. You feel that the administrator is totally out-of-line on this point, and you want to make a point that the way you provide care to your patients is up to you, NOT the administrator.

Training Tool #24

A question of priorities

TYPE: Role play – two physicians, Dr. Bush and Dr. Clinton

ESTIMATED TRAINING TIME: 30 minutes

THEMES: Conflict management, negotiation

OBJECTIVES:
➡ to identify ways to resolve disputes involving conflicting priorities;
➡ to provide practice in dealing with the substance of the conflict as well as the relationship.

MATERIALS NEEDED: Copies of the two roles for each dyad

PROCEDURE:
Ask participants to identify a partner. If there are an uneven number of participants, have the extra person serve as observer. Distribute the instructions for Drs. Bush and Clinton so that each person in the dyads is playing an opposing role. Announce that the group will have 15 minutes to complete the role play.

DEBRIEFING:
1 What are the issues in this scenario?
2 What did you do to address the strain in this relationship?
3 Did you assume that the doctors have a 50/50 split of the practice? If so, how would you have responded differently if Dr. Bush took home 35% and Dr. Clinton took 65%?
4 Did you resolve the conflict? If so, what strategies were most effective?
5 Did your solutions involve concessions by either or both parties? Compromises? Trade-offs? Creative solutions (in which both parties' needs are met without either losing on matters of greatest importance to them)?
6 Did any of the dyads reach a deadlock in this exercise? If so, what can be learned by those who reached a solution?

ROLE PLAY: A QUESTION OF PRIORITIES
CONFIDENTIAL INSTRUCTIONS

Dr. Bush

You realize that your physician colleague, Dr. Clinton, is very upset with you because you have refused to work evenings, do immunization clinics, or any of the extras that Dr. Clinton has been pressing you to do. Not only that, but you've told Dr. Clinton that you want to cut down on the amount of call you've been taking.

You have three very young children, and your spouse has been asking you to spend more time with the family, and you believe it's important to do that. Your colleague, Dr. Clinton, is more interested in building the practice, whereas you'd like reasonable hours and a balanced life. However, you are concerned that your relationship with Dr. Clinton has become increasingly strained.

ROLE PLAY: A QUESTION OF PRIORITIES
CONFIDENTIAL INSTRUCTIONS

Dr. Clinton

You are very upset with your colleague, Dr. Bush. You are trying to do everything you can to build up the practice – doing immunization clinics, after-hours care, and getting involved in the community. Unfortunately, however, you feel that you are doing this all on your own. Not only does Dr. Bush not want to do "the extras," he/she also wants to cut down on the amount of call. You don't like it when Dr. Bush says it's a matter of having a more balanced life; after all, you have a family too, and the less Dr. Bush helps out, the more you have to handle by yourself. You can feel the tensions building with Dr. Bush and it's now time to address the problem.

Perceptions that the
clinic coordinator
favors some staff
members over others

Preferential treatment

TYPE: Role play – front-office staff and clinic coordinator

ESTIMATED TRAINING TIME: 30 minutes

THEMES: Conflict management, difficult colleagues

OBJECTIVES:
➡ to identify the elements of conflict involving employer-employee relationships;
➡ to determine how health care leaders can resolve conflicts while improving management skills.

MATERIALS NEEDED: Copies of the two roles for each dyad

PROCEDURE:
Ask participants to identify a partner. If there are an uneven number of participants, have the extra person serve as observer. Distribute the instructions so that each person in the dyads is playing an opposing role. Announce a 15-minute time limit for the role play.

DEBRIEFING:
1 In your dyads, did the clinic coordinator admit to giving Jan preferential treatment? Why or why not?
2 Did the front-office staff member present the issue in a blaming way?
3 In addition to the need for the clinic coordinator to treat employees more equally, was the staff member's negativism addressed?
4 What other issues were raised?
5 What solutions were agreed upon?
6 Did the relationship improve after the discussion?

ROLE PLAY: PREFERENTIAL TREATMENT
CONFIDENTIAL INSTRUCTIONS

Front-Office Staff

You believe that the clinic coordinator is giving preferential treatment to one of your co-workers, Jan, who is on the same level as you on the organizational chart. Your immediate concern is that Jan got a better schedule than you for next month, even though you asked for that schedule first.

This isn't the only time you've taken the backseat. The clinic coordinator spends more time with Jan, and Jan seems to get more recognition than you during meetings. Because you see a pattern here, you're beginning to resent them both. You're about to discuss this matter with the clinic coordinator to seek more equitable treatment. You know you've been pretty negative about things lately, but you feel that you've been pushed in that direction.

ROLE PLAY: PREFERENTIAL TREATMENT
CONFIDENTIAL INSTRUCTIONS

Clinic Coordinator

You are about to meet with a member of your front-office staff who believes you've been giving preferential treatment to a co-worker, Jan, who is on her same level on the organizational chart.

You secretly admit to yourself that you HAVE shown favoritism to Jan on numerous occasions. For example, you gave Jan more flexibility in her schedule lately because she has some personal problems (i.e. day care issues and transportation problems getting to work). You frequently have lunch with Jan and sometimes even socialize after work. You tend to give Jan a great deal of recognition during staff meetings, but say very little about the staff member you will be meeting with today. You wonder if subconsciously, you're giving Jan better treatment because she is much less negative and such a delight to work with.

Two public health
officials don't see eye
to eye on priorities,
methods, and other
matters

Training Tool #26

A toxic situation

TYPE: Role play – epidemiologist and laboratory director

ESTIMATED TRAINING TIME: 45 minutes

THEMES: Conflict management, negotiation, difficult colleagues

OBJECTIVE:

➡ to identify ways to foster greater cooperation between two public health
professionals who find themselves in repeated conflicts.

MATERIALS NEEDED: A copy of the two roles for each dyad

PROCEDURE:

Ask participants to identify a partner. If there are an uneven number of participants, have
the extra person serve as observer. Distribute the instructions so that each person in the
dyads is given an opposing role. Tell participants they will have 25 minutes to complete
the role play.

DEBRIEFING:

1 What issues are involved in this series of conflicts?
2 Did you address (a) past conflicts and misunderstandings; (b) the need to consider the
   current request as a high priority; (c) the request to maintain communication during the
   testing of the influenza strain; and (d) the need for improved relations in the future?
3 What do you think has caused the communication problems between the director of
   epidemiology and the lab director?
4 Are the needs of each party valid?
5 What benefits will be realized by resolving this dispute? Were these benefits noted
   during the role play?
6 Did your dyad reach agreement during the discussion? If so, how? What strategies were
   most effective? If no agreements were reached, what caused the impasse?

ROLE PLAY: A TOXIC SITUATION
CONFIDENTIAL INSTRUCTIONS

Epidemiologist

As the director of epidemiology of your State Department of Health, you have grown increasingly concerned about a new strain of influenza that appears to be particularly dangerous to persons with compromised immune systems and the elderly. Around two dozen documented cases have shown up so far, and the strain is so virulent that you want to do something immediately. You and your team have obtained specimens that you need to have tested by the State's public health laboratory.

You are dreading this interaction with the lab because you have had problems working with them in the past. Once, for example, you asked the lab to process cultures for an outbreak in the southwestern part of the state, but they did different tests than those you requested. You got the results you needed, but don't understand why they didn't follow instructions. Another time, it took them quite a while to get results back to you, even though you stressed – verbally and in writing, in the strongest possible terms – that your test was the HIGHEST possible priority. On a third occasion, laboratory scientists said they would like to provide training to your team of epidemiologists so that they would know how to give them good samples. How insulting! After all, you are not aware of any problems that the lab had with samples taken by your team.

After each of these instances, you met with the laboratory director to try to work things out so that the same problems wouldn't recur in the future. In your opinion, those meetings were a complete waste of time. The lab director was quite defensive, and you said you were tired of all the excuses. No solutions were reached at those meetings.

In addition to being very supportive of your epidemiology team, you take your job quite seriously. You have been under great pressure from the Director of the State Health Department to get moving more quickly on your investigations and you don't like being blamed when you feel that the lab is responsible for the slowdown.

It's time for your meeting with the lab director. You plan to make your case that testing the new influenza strain needs to be a MAJOR priority. To ensure that things run smoothly, you would like to communicate with the lab on an ongoing basis for the duration of this project.

ROLE PLAY: A TOXIC SITUATION
CONFIDENTIAL INSTRUCTIONS

Laboratory Director

You are about to meet with the director of epidemiology of the State Department of Health, and you are certainly not looking forward to this encounter! Every time the epidemiologists ask you to do something for them, they don't ask, they TELL. They seem to think that whatever is a priority to them must be the lab's priority too. You've tried to educate them about the lab's many pressures when you met with the director of epidemiology in the past, but when you pointed out the increasing demands on the lab, they said it was nothing but excuses. You've also offered a training session for them on how to provide clean samples, but they refused, saying they were insulted and that they know what they're doing. Don't they realize it's a course you offer to everyone you work with?

Above all, you hate it when the director of epidemiology complains about the lab, and that seems to be his/her favorite pastime. Once, the epi-director got very angry because the lab didn't process cultures for an outbreak in the manner requested. Another complaint was that you didn't get results back to them for quite a while, even though they expected results immediately. You admit it: both of those charges are completely true! The lab DID use a different method on one of the tests because you knew of a test that was just as accurate but less expensive. And yes, the lab DID delay on getting results of another test back to them. It's not an excuse when you point out all the demands placed on your lab; you simply don't have the resources to do everything that everyone wants exactly when they want it. With a limited number of personnel, there are times when you can't do more than one or two projects at a time.

Whatever the director of epidemiology requests today, you are sure it will be presented as "the highest possible priority." You doubt that anything will be more important than what the lab is focusing on right now: a cluster of *E coli* that has already infected hundreds of persons. Your staff is now working double shifts, so other projects will have to wait. You especially want to cut down on meetings and phone calls because you and your staff have to be completely focused on getting all the work done without so many interruptions.

It's time now for your meeting.

The Divisions' dilemma

TYPE: Role play – representatives of the following Divisions in a State health department:
➡ Communicable Diseases
➡ Children's Health
➡ Regulation

ESTIMATED TRAINING TIME: 60 minutes

THEMES: Conflict management, negotiation, difficult colleagues

OBJECTIVE:
➡ to identify ways to resolve disputes laden with power struggles, past differences, and personality conflicts.

MATERIALS NEEDED: Copies of the instruction sheet for all participants

PROCEDURE:
Ask participants to divide into groups of three. If there are extra persons, ask them to serve as observer or double up on a role with one of the others. Distribute the instruction sheet and ask each person in the triad to assume a different role. Tell the group they will have 35 minutes to complete the role play. Note that the goal of the meeting will be to determine how the three Divisions might work together on this project. Also mention that if an agreement cannot be determined, the funding for this project is likely to be rescinded.

DEBRIEFING:
1 Did your triad resolve this matter successfully? Which Division would take the lead? What other issues were discussed?
2 What strategies worked best for bringing the group to consensus? Or, if no agreement was reached, what happened?
3 What was the compelling reason for these Divisions to come to agreement? What are the perils of not working together effectively?
4 How have the problems in these Divisions' past relationships affected this discussion?
5 How did your group address personality conflicts?

ROLE PLAY: THE DIVISION'S DILEMMA

The State Department of Health has received federal funds to develop licensing standards for day care centers throughout the State. A huge sum of money is involved and the project will have a high national profile. The federal agency providing the funds has mandated the collaboration of three Divisions on this project: Communicable Diseases, Children's Health, and Regulation. There is great pressure on the three Divisions to work together effectively on this project, but unfortunately the three Divisions do not have a good track record of getting along. Today, representatives of the three Divisions will meet to determine how they can best work together on this project and which Division will take the lead. Issues they will need to consider are as follows:

▶ **Communicable Diseases:** This Division will be responsible for standards related to the prevention and management of dozens of communicable diseases that are reportable under State law – everything from head lice to pertussis. Communicable Diseases believes that it should take the lead because, due to a previous career, the director of this Division has more experience with day care centers than the other two directors. The Division believes that Regulation doesn't have the knowledge about the subject matter that is necessary to lead the project, and that Children's Health shouldn't lead because they historically have not shared information or data to the extent that they should and are not good at collaborating.

▶ **Children's Health:** For this project, Children's Health will write standards for children with special needs, product safety, and all other matters to protect children that are not related to communicable disease. This Division wants to take the lead because they feel that their responsibilities are much greater in scope than the other two Divisions and that most of the standards will come from them. They believe that Communicable Diseases does not have the capability of taking the lead; after all, they frequently get off track, often requesting information on matters that do not concern them. They also believe that the director of Communicable Diseases thinks that she's an expert on everything and is very difficult to work with. Several employees in this Division also have a major personality conflicts with representatives from the Division of Regulation and see them as "control freaks." The ones they've had problems with the most are those attending today's meeting.

▶ **Regulation:** This Division believes it should take the lead on this project and make most or all of the major decisions without having to consult with Children's Health or Communicable Diseases. The Division of Regulation would be happy to consult with the other two Divisions as necessary, but doesn't want to have every decision stalled by the squabbling between Children's Health and Communicable Diseases. They feel that getting the job done expeditiously is much more important than working together and that they are best suited for a coordinating role.

Dispute on expanding
a residency
program's facility in a
cost-effective way

Training Tool #28

Expansion plans

TYPE: Role play – Residency Program Director and Hospital Administrator

ESTIMATED TRAINING TIME: 60 minutes

THEMES: Conflict management, negotiation

OBJECTIVES:
➡ resolve a multi-issue dispute in ways that address short-term and long-term needs;
➡ to demonstrate the importance of understanding the perspectives and needs of each party.

MATERIALS NEEDED: Copies of the two roles for each dyad

PROCEDURE:
Ask participants to select a partner. If there are an uneven number of participants, ask the extra person to serve as observer or double up on a role with one of the others. Distribute the instructions so that each person in the dyads is playing a different role. Give the group 35 minutes to complete the role play and then bring them back together for an all-group discussion.

DEBRIEFING:
1 What are the issues in this dispute?
2 Is the Residency Director truly unconcerned with the financial aspects of his/her request? Is the Administrator not fully appreciating the program's desire for future growth?
3 What are the two parties' mutual interests and needs?
4 What solutions did your dyad suggest? What will be the long-term effects of those solutions?
5 Will the solutions have an impact on other residencies and units within the medical center? If so, what?
6 What strategies were most effective in convincing the other party of your character's needs?

ROLE PLAY: EXPANSION PLANS
CONFIDENTIAL INSTRUCTIONS

Residency Program Director

Established 10 years ago, the Family Medicine Residency Program at St. Otherplace Medical Center has been quite successful and now trains a total of 18 residents. You have been the director since the program's inception.

Currently, the residency has a total of 18 000 square feet on the 12th floor of the medical center. You are becoming increasingly concerned that the program has outgrown its existing space. Your residents are currently overloaded with patients, the clinic's waiting room is overcrowded, and your faculty members are being stretched to their limits.

Today, you will meet with the Administrator of St. Otherplace Medical Center to discuss the program's expansion needs. Considered as a "visionary" by your colleagues, you have many dreams of what the program could achieve, and you believe strongly that the program has a tremendous, but as yet unrealized, potential. Your first choice is to build a new family medicine clinic with a ground floor entrance. You would like to at least double the space to 36 000 square feet. When you checked with several sources on the cost for this new building, the lowest cost was $4 million. However, since the new building would attract many more patients, you don't see that as a problem.

Another option is to remodel some of the existing space at the medical center. However, this is less appealing to you because there still is no ground-floor space available. In the past, the administrator mentioned the possibility of remodeling the 13th floor. The cost of this would be $2 million. Sure, there would be savings on the front end, but you believe that the administrator should see the long-term benefits of a new facility.

Also, you would like to add two new faculty members and six additional residents. With a new building, you believe that it will be an easy matter to recruit the needed faculty and new residents. This will help you to increase the practice's patient population, train more residents for rural practice, and meet even more of the community's needs. (Because of several new industries in town, local physicians often complain about heavy patient loads.)

In addition to meeting many of the community's needs, you are proud of the fact that your program has served as a key revenue source that has kept the medical center solvent through its inpatient admissions. You would like to get the administrator's commitment and support for your plans.

ROLE PLAY: EXPANSION PLANS
CONFIDENTIAL INSTRUCTIONS

Administrator

You have been the Administrator of St. Otherplace Medical Center for the past five years. Five years before you arrived, the family medicine residency program was established. With a quite successful record of accomplishments, the program now has a total of 18 residents.

Currently, the residency has a total of 18 000 square feet on the medical center's 12th floor (which is virtually all of the usable space on that floor). You acknowledge that the program has outgrown its existing space. The question is how to help the program to acquire the space it needs, while still being fiscally responsible.

Today, you will meet with the Director of the Family Medicine Residency Program to seek a solution. You think it would be ludicrous to build a new facility when there are two floors in the medical center that are not being used to full capacity. The third floor now houses a unit that is likely to be eliminated as a cost-cutting measure, and the 13th floor is currently vacant. Renovating either of these floors would cost $2 million. If you approved the construction of a new building, you're sure the cost would be at least double that amount.

You have a feeling that the Director of the Family Medicine Residency Program will ask for the moon, which is very frustrating to you. For as long as you've been an administrator, it has seemed that doctors just don't get it; they don't understand financial constraints that you must deal with, and that several departments and other residencies are pressuring you for expenditures as well.

As a practical matter, you'd like to start by having the existing faculty and residents expand their hours. If they need more space for their current needs, you will commit to renovating existing space. However, if they want to expand their faculty and resident positions, you think that should wait. In addition to the fact that you've just put a freeze on new hiring, adding more faculty will increase the program's educational costs. Of course, the doctors don't even consider that!

You aren't totally opposed to taking reasonable risks, and you'd like to be helpful to the program since it's been a very good revenue source for the medical center. Nevertheless, the Director of the Family Medicine Residency is known as a "big dreamer" and you believe it's up to you to point out the realities of the political climate and the uncertainties about future federal funding. You don't want to damper the director's enthusiasm, but you do want to convince him/her to "get real."

Dispute on whether
a social worker
or nurse educator
should run a project

FamCare: a difference in perspectives

TYPE: Role play – two directors within a state health department:

➡ Division of Family Health Services

➡ Maternal-Child Health (MCH) Education Branch

ESTIMATED TRAINING TIME: 30 minutes

THEMES: Conflict management, negotiation

OBJECTIVES:

➡ to understand the dynamics of intra-agency conflict;

➡ to apply conflict management strategies to resolve differences and arrive at the best solution for the organization.

MATERIALS NEEDED: Copies of the following page for each participant

PROCEDURE:

Ask participants to select a partner and ask each person in the dyad to play an opposing role. If there are an uneven number of participants, ask the extra person to serve as observer or double up on a role with one of the others. Give the group 15 minutes to complete the role play; then bring them back together for an all-group discussion.

DEBRIEFING:

1 Did each dyad reach a consensus about how to handle this dilemma? If so, what strategies were most effective in resolving the matter? If not, what caused the deadlock?

2 What type of professional did your dyad decide to hire: a social worker or nurse educator? What was the rationale? Did the fact that FamCare will be managed by the MCH/Health Education Branch influence your decision?

3 Should the Division of Family Health Services have greater weight in this decision because of its position in the organizational hierarchy? Why or why not?

4 What dynamics in this intra-agency conflict contributed to the way in which the situation was resolved?

5 Thinking a year ahead, will the solutions reached by your dyad be likely to contribute to additional conflicts in the future? If so, what? How can such conflicts be avoided?

6 If you also did Training Tool #27, how did your discussion about which party should lead vary from that situation to this one?

ROLE PLAY: FAMCARE: A DIFFERENCE IN PERSPECTIVES

In the very near future, a new program (which has been nicknamed "FamCare") will be initiated in the State health department; the program has been designed to promote primary care for families with young children. The program will be under the State's Division of Family Health Services, but it will be located in the Maternal and Child Health (MCH)/Health Education Branch.

The program is ready to be implemented, except for one major glitch: there is a dispute regarding the type of professional that should be hired to direct the new program.

▶ **Division of Family Health Services:** The Chief of Family Health Services strongly believes that a social worker should be in charge because of social workers' training and experience in family dynamics and health behaviors. His/her staff agrees; they also contend that their opinions should have greater weight in this decision because the Division of Family Health Services is above MCH/Health Education in the organizational hierarchy.

▶ **Maternal and Child Health/Health Education Branch:** Those in the MCH/Health Education Branch believe just as strongly that a nurse educator should fill this position in order to provide the necessary clinical perspective. They believe their views should take precedence because the new person who is hired will be physically located in MCH/Health Education, and the entire FamCare program will be managed through the MCH/Health Education Branch.

The Director of Public Health could have just made a decision about this issue one way or the other, but thinks it would be better if this issue were addressed by the parties who will be most affected. The director has asked the heads of both groups to meet to discuss the pros and cons of each option and to try to reach a consensus today so that the program can get underway. The Personnel Department will create a job description for this position, but cannot do so until there is a final decision about which discipline should be hired.

Whether case
managers or parent
consultants should
help children with
special needs

Changing roles

TYPE: Role play
➥ Case manager
➥ Parent consultant

ESTIMATED TRAINING TIME: 30 minutes

THEMES: Conflict management, negotiation

OBJECTIVE:
➥ to provide experience in dealing with a conflict involving mutual ownership of responsibilities.

MATERIALS NEEDED: Copies of the following page for each participant

PROCEDURE:
Ask participants to select a partner. If there are an uneven number of participants, ask the extra person to serve as observer, double up on a role with one of the characters in their group, or play the role of the Director of the Maternal and Child Health Division. There is one instruction sheet for all participants. Assign each individual to play an opposing role. Tell the group they will have 15 minutes to conduct the role play; then bring them back together for an all-group discussion.

DEBRIEFING:
1 What arguments by the case managers and parent consultants were most effective? Which were least effective?
2 How did your dyad handle the issue of cost-effectiveness? Training and qualifications? Relationships with the families?
3 Did the parent consultants' threats to resign have a bearing on this case? Why or why not?
4 What were your mutual interests?
5 Did your dyad develop a creative solution to this conflict, i.e. one in which some if not all of each parties' needs are met? If so, what?

ROLE PLAY: CHANGING ROLES

Six months ago, the State Health Department's Division of Maternal and Child Health (MCH) hired 15 parent consultants to handle many of the direct contacts with families of children with special needs. Since that time, the case managers, who have been doing this work for the past several years, have become very upset. In addition to losing what they consider to be one of the most fulfilling parts of their jobs, the case managers believe that hiring the parent consultants is a "professional slap in the face." As one case manager stated, "How can someone with five days of training provide the same kind of assistance that I can with my advanced degrees and 10 years of experience in maternal and child health?"

When the parent consultants found out about the case managers' complaints, they became rather defensive. The parent consultants believe that they are doing a good job and that since they are the parents of children with special needs themselves, they can identify with these families in a way that the case managers cannot. Regardless, the parent consultants are extremely disheartened that the case managers have been so vocal about their complaints, and some are so upset that they have threatened to resign.

The Director of Maternal and Child Health understands each party's concerns, but has been trying to make this work out because (a) this program is saving money; (b) it's possible to reach more families with special needs with the assistance of the parent consultants; and (c) this allows the case managers to spend more of their time on the most intensive and complicated cases.

In order to address this conflict and work out some creative solutions, the Director has invited one representative of the case managers and one representative of the parent consultants to a meeting. All parties have agreed to abide by whatever the two of them work out.

The recalcitrant resident

TYPE: Role play – Chief Resident and Director of the Family Medicine Residency Program

ESTIMATED TRAINING TIME: 60 minutes

THEMES: Conflict management, negotiation

OBJECTIVE:

➡ to demonstrate effective ways of dealing with a multi-issue conflict.

MATERIALS NEEDED: Copies of the two roles for each dyad

PROCEDURE:

Ask participants to select a partner. If there are an uneven number of participants, ask the extra person to serve as observer or double up on a role with one of the others. Distribute the instructions so that each person is playing a different role. Tell the group they will have 35 minutes to conduct the role play. After this time, bring everyone back for an all-group discussion.

DEBRIEFING:

1 Were all three of the residents' concerns addressed during this meeting? Did any issues fall through the cracks?

2 To what extent was each party making an effort to listen and understand the other's positions and interests?

3 What techniques did each person use to uncover the other party's real needs?

4 Did power differences play a role in the resolution of this dispute? If so, how?

5 Were your solutions satisfactory to each party? What strategies or techniques made such solutions possible?

6 Assuming that some or most of the dyads had different results, what accounts for those differences?

ROLE PLAY: THE RECALCITRANT RESIDENT
CONFIDENTIAL INSTRUCTIONS

Chief Resident

You are the Chief Resident of the Family Medicine Residency Program at Wayout Hospital. You are currently in your second year. Counting you, there are 18 residents in your program.

When you came to the program, you knew that the program director was a big proponent of rural practice and OB training, including complicated procedures. At the time, you hadn't yet decided where to practice, so these factors were not a deterrent. You were attracted to the program at Wayout because of the program director's excellent reputation, and also because Wayout is near the hometown of your spouse. While some residents came to the program because of the rural and OB emphasis, most residents came to the program for reasons similar to yours.

At a residents' meeting with your program director about a week ago, many of the residents voiced their complaints regarding these issues:

▶ **Rural Practice:** Since only 5 of the 18 residents at your program plan on entering rural practice, the rest of them (including you) would like to eliminate (or shorten) the eight weeks you are required to spend on rural rotation. Although there were four other residents who expressed an interest in rural practice when they came to the program, you don't think they will end up going into it.

▶ **OB Training:** Only the five residents who plan on rural practice want to be trained in complicated OB. The rest of you don't plan on including that in your future practices for a variety of reasons: (a) not interested in it/don't plan on ever using it; (b) professional liability; (c) the belief that their time could be better spent in other areas; and (d) concerns about being trained in OB by family medicine faculty rather than by OBs. (OB is currently taught by two family physician faculty members, and back-up is provided by three OBs on the Wayout Hospital staff. The OBs have not been very nice to the residents, and one in particular has been very difficult to deal with.)

▶ **Balance:** Most residents believe that the program's demands on their time are too great, and believe they should have more time off. Many of the residents have young children, and believe the program should be more concerned with "quality of life" issues.

On a more basic level, you believe that the program should train residents in accordance with the types of practice they are planning – not based on the biases of the program director!

When you tried to discuss these issues with the program director last week during the residents' meeting, the program director seemed to get defensive, explained his/her views, and asked the residents to think these matters over. This morning, you asked for a meeting to try to work things out. The residents have told you that unless there's more flexibility on the program director's part, they want you to speak to Dr. Yessen Deedee, Wayout Hospital's Director of Medical Education, and/or Ms. Mary Lou Nobucks, the hospital administrator, to try to get support.

You are also aware that five of the residents are strongly supportive of the program's emphasis, believe that the program director is doing a wonderful job, and think that the rest of you should not be engaged in all this opposition. These five didn't even want you to have the meeting with the program director today.

Your meeting with the program director is right now, and you are now knocking on the program director's door.

ROLE PLAY: THE RECALCITRANT RESIDENT
CONFIDENTIAL INSTRUCTIONS

Family Medicine Residency Program Director

You became the Director of the Family Medicine Residency Program at Wayout Hospital five years ago. The City of Wayout is located in a fairly rural area of the State.

All along, your key priorities for the program have been to (a) encourage rural practice, and (b) ensure that your family medicine residents learn how to perform basic and advanced obstetrical procedures so that they will be better equipped to handle all types of situations if they choose to engage in rural practice. These views are strongly supported by Wayout Hospital's Director of Medical Education, Dr. Yessen Deedee. The hospital administrator, Ms. Mary Lou Nobucks, is willing to go along with any emphasis for the program that you and Dr. Deedee decide as long as your decisions do not cost the hospital extra money.

You feel so strongly about rural and OB training for your residents that you have even been quoted in some of the local and regional papers about your views. You have also made a big point about your program's emphasis on OB and rural practice in the new promotional brochures you developed for your program this year. These brochures have been widely distributed.

Currently, two highly skilled family physicians on your faculty are providing the OB training to your residents. Three OBs on the hospital staff are providing back-up, albeit somewhat reluctantly.

You realize that not all of your residents are going to go into rural practice and/or include OB in their practices, but you believe that it's essential to teach the full range of family medicine. You also believe that residents should have exposure to rural practice and the full range of OB so that they can make more informed decisions.

During the past five years, between 50% and 55% of your residents went into rural practice. This year, however, only 5 of your 18 residents have expressed an interest in rural practice. (Four others had originally expressed an interest but don't seem committed to it.) Although some of your residents have complained in recent months about your insistence on training in complicated OB, you were not aware of the intensity of their feelings until you attended a meeting of the residents that was held last week. With a few exceptions, most of the residents complained about being trained in complicated OB, having to endure eight weeks of rural rotation, and not having enough time for their personal lives. (When you were a resident, you worked many more hours than they are putting in now, and you have little tolerance for residents who keep complaining about not having enough balance between their personal and professional lives.) One of the residents even had the nerve to complain that their OB training was by family physicians rather than OBs! During that meeting, you tried to explain your views to the residents, but you still met a great deal of resistance. You asked the residents to think about your views, and left that meeting very upset.

This morning, you had a call from the chief resident who has asked for a meeting to try to work out your differences, and you agreed to meet. It's now time for that meeting, and the chief resident is knocking at your door.

Training Tool #32

Shifting resources in a State health agency

TYPE: Role play – representatives of middle management and senior management in a Maternal and Child Health (MCH) Division of a State health department

ESTIMATED TRAINING TIME: 30 minutes

THEMES: Conflict management, negotiation

OBJECTIVES:

➡ to demonstrate that what may seem to be a single issue conflict actually has numerous layers, each of which needs to be resolved;

➡ to show the importance of dealing with issues by "unbundling" them into their smallest, most manageable parts.

MATERIALS NEEDED: Copies of the two roles for members of each group

PROCEDURE:

Ask participants to break into groups of four or five. It does not matter if there are an uneven number of participants; just be sure that approximately half of each group are assigned to the role of senior management, and the other half are middle management. Give the group 15 minutes to conduct the role play; then conduct an all-group discussion.

DEBRIEFING:

1   How did the needs of senior management differ from those of middle management?
2   What issues are involved in this case, in addition to the possibility of reducing the number of clerical staff? How were those issues handled by your group? Did any of the issues fall through the cracks?
3   Was the morale issue addressed?
4   Did your dyad address middle management's desire to provide more input? What about managing the workload?
5   How was this conflict resolved? Were each party's needs met?
6   Did the way in which the conflict was handled improve relationships between middle and senior management?

ROLE PLAY: SHIFTING RESOURCES IN A STATE HEALTH AGENCY
CONFIDENTIAL INSTRUCTIONS

Middle Management

There is a rumor that senior management in the Maternal and Child Health (MCH) Division is seriously considering cutting the clerical staff from 10 persons to 6 in order to have enough money to hire a new nurse practitioner for the Division. The rumor is true. The plan is to hire the nurse practitioner for a senior management position.

You and your colleagues in middle management have been quite upset since hearing this rumor (which you were not consulted about) and morale among middle managers is at an all-time low. You've asked senior management for a meeting to discuss this issue, and senior management agreed.

You're aware that the Division budget is exceptionally tight and that there is a tremendous need for another nurse practitioner in the Division. Nevertheless, you are concerned about this matter for three reasons.

▶ You are tired of senior management making decisions without getting middle management's input in advance.

▶ Even with 10 clerical staff, it takes far too long to get back your paperwork as it is; you expect even greater delays with only 6 clerical staff.

▶ If a new nurse practitioner is hired, that will increase the workload of clerical staff even more. This doesn't make sense as there will be fewer clerical staff to do the work!

ROLE PLAY: SHIFTING RESOURCES IN A STATE HEALTH AGENCY
CONFIDENTIAL INSTRUCTIONS

Senior Management

There is a rumor floating around that you and your colleagues in senior management are seriously considering cutting the clerical staff from 10 persons to 6 in order to have enough money to hire a new nurse practitioner for the division. The rumor is true. The nurse practitioner would be hired for a senior management position.

Middle management in the Maternal and Child Health (MCH) Division is quite upset since they have not been consulted about the proposed cut in clerical staff, so you and your colleagues agreed to meet with them to assuage their concerns. The middle managers you'll meet with today already know that the Division budget is exceptionally tight and that there is a tremendous need for another nurse practitioner in the Division.

You believe that the Division's greatest priority is to get another nurse practitioner on staff to help divide up the senior management's workload. You and other senior managers are now working so much overtime that your families barely recognize you anymore. Tensions are extremely high, morale among senior managers is at an all-time low, and you and the other senior managers have decided to do something about it. After all, getting a more equitable distribution of the workload should obviously supersede the problem of having paperwork take a little longer every now and then.

Special delivery

TYPE: Role play – leadership teams representing family medicine and obstetrics-gynecology

ESTIMATED TRAINING TIME: 60 minutes

THEMES: Conflict management, negotiation

OBJECTIVES:

➡ to show the dynamics and issues involved in inter-specialty conflict;

➡ to demonstrate ways to resolve conflicts involving two specialties performing the same procedures.

MATERIALS NEEDED: Copies of the two roles distributed evenly in each small group

PROCEDURE:

Ask participants to form small groups. Distribute the instructions so that approximately half of the group is playing each role. After 35 minutes for the role play, engage in an all-group discussion.

DEBRIEFING:

1 What are the issues involved in this conflict? Are the issues about turf? Dollars? Quality? Principles? Something else?
2 In terms of this conflict, what is the impact of the OBs' concerns about providing backup to family physicians doing deliveries?
3 How did your dyad handle the conflicting points about qualifications?
4 How does your profession or discipline affect the way you view this matter?
5 How do the concerns of the two specialties differ? What are their mutual needs and interests?
6 What solutions were reached in this conflict?

ROLE PLAY: SPECIAL DELIVERY
CONFIDENTIAL INSTRUCTIONS

Leadership Team: Obstetrics and Gynecology

FabuCare is the largest multi-specialty group in the state. When the plan was established in 1980, obstetricians-gynecologists were far outnumbered by family physicians. During those early years, family physicians practiced a broad range of obstetrical procedures. Although some family physicians no longer are interested in OB due to lifestyle concerns and liability insurance, there are still many of the older family physicians and several recent residency graduates that enjoy doing obstetrics.

In recent years, the plan has dramatically increased its number of OBs. This year, you and other obstetricians-gynecologists have been speaking up about your belief that family physicians should no longer be doing normal vaginal deliveries. Since obstetricians-gynecologists are called in for back-up, and because professional liability insurance for obstetrics has increased dramatically, your colleagues believe that it is not a good idea to have family physicians perform normal vaginal deliveries when obstetricians-gynecologists are available to do so.

You and your colleagues believe strongly that deliveries have better outcomes when they are done by the physicians who perform these procedures most frequently. You do not see this as a freedom of choice issue; you see this as a quality issue. You also do not want family physicians to be managing complications when OBs are available; neither do you want them to do VBACs (vaginal births after caesarean). There is much more disagreement among obstetricians-gynecologists about the types of pregnancy care that family physicians are capable of providing. Some believe that family physicians can provide care for patients with mild pre-eclampsia and pre-existing hypertension; others do not.

FabuCare officials believe this is a practice issue that should be worked out between OB and family medicine. They plan to make the decision themselves about this matter if the two specialties do not come up with a solution. If that happens, you have no idea how their decision would turn out.

ROLE PLAY: SPECIAL DELIVERY
CONFIDENTIAL INSTRUCTIONS

Leadership Team: Family Medicine

FabuCare is the largest multi-specialty group in the State. When the plan was started in 1980, there were more family physicians than other types of specialists. During those early years, family physicians practiced a broad range of obstetrical procedures. While some family physicians are no longer interested in OB due to lifestyle concerns and professional liability insurance, there are still many older doctors and quite a few recent residency graduates who enjoy the obstetrical component of their practice and feel very strongly about maintaining their competency in this area.

In recent years, the plan has dramatically increased its number of OBs. This year, the obstetricians have raised concerns that family physicians should no longer be doing normal vaginal deliveries. The OBs, who are called in for back-up, believe that it is not a good idea to have family physicians perform normal vaginal deliveries when they are available to do so.

You and your colleagues believe strongly that family physicians should be able to perform the procedures for which they are qualified and trained. In fact, you believe that family physicians should be able to do any type of pregnancy care in accordance with their demonstrated current competence. Even those who do not choose to do OB believe that others should have the freedom of choice to do so or not. You have seen numerous studies showing that family physicians provide high-quality obstetrical care, so you do not believe that quality should be an issue.

In a broader sense, you and your colleagues in family medicine are concerned that your scope of practice in managed health care is being eroded a little more each year. There is also a fear that, because FabuCare is a prominent provider within the State, the role of family physicians within this plan may have an effect on the role of family physicians elsewhere.

FabuCare officials believe this is a practice issue that should be worked out between OB and family medicine. They have said that they will make the decision themselves about this matter if the two specialties do not come up with a solution. If that happens, you have no idea how their decision will turn out.

Training Tool #34

Working hand-in-hand

TYPE: Role play – the Chair of the Plastic Surgery Division and the Chair of the Department of Orthopedics at Complexity Medical Center

ESTIMATED TRAINING TIME: 45 minutes

THEMES: Conflict management, negotiation

OBJECTIVES:

➡ to demonstrate the dynamics and issues involved in an inter-specialty conflict;

➡ to show how an organizational conflict involving limited resources can be resolved successfully.

MATERIALS NEEDED: A copy of the following page for all participants

PROCEDURE:

Ask participants to select a partner and to determine who will play the role of Chair of the Plastic Surgery Division and who will play the Chair of the Department of Orthopedics. If there are an uneven number of participants, ask the extra person to serve as observer or double up on a role with one of the others. After giving the dyads 20–25 minutes to resolve the conflict, bring them back together for an all-group discussion.

DEBRIEFING:

1 Given that only one hand surgeon can be hired, does this situation have to be resolved in a win-lose manner? How can this be a win-win for plastic surgery and orthopedics?

2 How was the situation resolved by your dyad?

3 How did your dyad handle specific issues you were asked to consider, such as training, medical records, and space?

4 If your dyad reached a deadlock and decided to let the Dean resolve this issue, what were the roadblocks to reaching a consensus?

ROLE PLAY: WORKING HAND-IN-HAND

Complexity Medical Center is one of the largest and most prestigious academic medical centers in the region. However, not unlike many other medical centers, revenues during the past three years have been particularly tight.

The Division of Plastic Surgery and the Department of Orthopedics is each in the process of recruiting a new hand surgeon. Until now, neither has consulted with the other on their recruitment efforts. Both the Division and the Department maintain that they need their own hand surgeon in order to keep the revenues in their own areas and to have attractive residency training programs.

Not counting the residents and fellows from each specialty, a total of five surgeons are currently performing hand surgery at Complexity Medical Center. The four hand surgeons from the Department of Orthopedics have been particularly busy during the past year or so, and have insisted on receiving additional assistance. The one surgeon performing hand surgeries from the Plastic Surgery Division is planning to retire next month. (Currently, each surgeon performing hand surgery is going to the OR about two to three times a week.)

When the Dean heard that the Plastic Surgery Division and the Department of Orthopedics were both trying to recruit a hand surgeon, he got very upset. He called in both of the Chairs to tell them that, although there was plenty of volume to justify hiring one hand surgeon, two would be too many considering the anticipated number of hand surgery patients. He suggested that the two Chairs get together to determine which specialty should do the hiring, and how to handle other considerations such as training programs, medical records, and space.

If the Chairs reach a deadlock, however, the Dean said that he would make the decision for them.

Negotiation – bargaining skills

Future uses of negotiation skills

TYPE: Introductory discussion

ESTIMATED TRAINING TIME: 15 minutes

THEME: Negotiation

OBJECTIVE:

➥ to show the numerous ways participants will use negotiation skills throughout their careers.

MATERIALS NEEDED: Flip chart

PROCEDURE:

To introduce the topic, ask the group how they currently use negotiating/bargaining skills in their health care careers, and how they plan to use these skills in the future. List the responses on a flip chart.

Likely responses include:

➥ negotiating treatment plans with patients;

➥ dealing with conflicts with colleagues and others;

➥ managed care and other types of contracts;

➥ employee agreements;

➥ reimbursement arrangements with third-party payers;

➥ partnership or group practice agreements;

➥ buying, leasing or selling arrangements (e.g., for equipment or computer systems);

➥ length-of-stay arrangements with case managers;

➥ the sale of a practice;

➥ mergers and acquisitions, etc.

DEBRIEFING:

Next, ask participants what they would most like to learn about this vital skill. Record the responses to ensure that these topics are addressed in the course.

Considering the
needs of persons
who are not
physically present at
the negotiating table

Training Tool #36

The empty chair

TYPE: Introductory discussion

ESTIMATED TRAINING TIME: 15 minutes

THEME: Negotiation

OBJECTIVE:

➡ to underscore the importance of considering the needs, interests, and perspectives of those who are affected by negotiated decisions, but are not present to represent themselves.

MATERIALS NEEDED: None

PROCEDURE:

Read the following descriptions of health care negotiations to participants, and note that you will ask them what these cases have in common:

➡ Physicians, nurses, and administrators of a local hospital discuss ways to improve cardiology services.

➡ Physicians, nurses, and physician assistants discuss ways to handle a difficult patient.

➡ A physician and a case manager at a managed care organization discuss their differing preferences regarding a patient's length of stay in the hospital.

➡ A physician talks to a family about whether to remove their terminally ill daughter's feeding tube.

Give the group a hint: "You know who is at the negotiating table. Who *isn't* there?"

DEBRIEFING:

Point out that this discussion is not to say that the patient should be present in these instances, but rather that the person who is most affected by the decisions is normally not there to offer their wishes and perspectives. In fact, one might say that the most important person in this discussion is the one in the "empty chair." Then ask:

1 What are the best ways to remind ourselves to consider the person in the empty chair?

2 What is the likely effect of considering the empty chair in our health care negotiations?

Negotiation self-test

TYPE: Self-test

ESTIMATED TRAINING TIME: 30 minutes

THEME: Negotiation

OBJECTIVES:
➡ to identify participants' negotiation styles: hard, soft, or principled;
➡ to explain the benefits of using a principled style of negotiation – the style that is most conducive to win-win outcomes.

MATERIALS NEEDED: A copy of the self-test on the following pages: the self-test (distribute this first); and the score sheet (distribute this after participants have taken the test)

PROCEDURE:
Distribute a copy of the self-test to each participant and give them 10–15 minutes to fill it out. Because people tend to behave somewhat differently at home than at work, tell participants that they should consider their negotiation tendencies in terms of their work. Also advise them to select the answer for each question that best describes their tendencies rather than the answer they think is "correct."

DEBRIEFING:
After participants have completed filling out their self-test, distribute the score sheet and ask them to circle their response for each question. The heading with the most circles indicates their predominant style. As noted on the score sheet, "A" responses represent a "soft" negotiating style, "B" is "hard," and "C" is "principled."

Point out that the *hard* negotiation style is a winner-take-all ("I win, you lose") approach, which focuses on the issue, but does not take into consideration the other parties' needs and does not foster relationship-building as much as the other two styles. (If anyone says that they do not care about relationship-building during a negotiation, point out that they may need to negotiate with the other party again in the future, and if so, the other party may decide to retaliate – or may decide not to negotiate with them at all. Another point is that good relationships normally lead to better deals.)

Those with a predominantly *soft* negotiation style are apt to give the greatest attention to the relationship, while not giving nearly enough attention to the substance of the negotiation. These negotiators typically make too many unnecessary concessions and are less likely to get their real needs met. It is most likely that those using this style will achieve an "I lose-you win" outcome.

The most preferred style is the principled negotiation style, also known as "interest bargaining." This is the style in which a win-win outcome is most likely. It is neither hard nor soft; it is open and direct. Principled negotiators focus on both their own interests as well as those of the other party.

Note: For more information about the differences between these styles, see *Getting to Yes: Negotiating Agreement without Giving In*, by Roger Fisher, William Ury, and Bruce Patton.

Negotiation self-test[2]

Which of the following statements most closely characterizes your negotiation style?

(Note: Be sure to select the response that is most true about your style, not the one you think you're "supposed" to choose.)

_____ 1 **I tend to view the other parties in a negotiation as:**
   a. Worthy opponents who are there to make the best deal they can for themselves
   b. Potential friends who are there to address our mutual interests
   c. Neither friends nor adversaries

_____ 2 **In a negotiation, I usually rely more on:**
   a. My people skills
   b. The strategies and thinking I have done to prepare for the negotiation
   c. My experience and gut instincts

_____ 3 **In regard to "trust" in a negotiation:**
   a. It should not affect the negotiation one way or the other
   b. It is best to be cautious about the other party until you know who you're dealing with
   c. It is best to trust other people up front until you are given reason to feel otherwise

_____ 4 **In most of my negotiations, I feel that:**
   a. I need the other party more than they need me, even though I won't let them know that
   b. The other party needs me as much as I need them, whether or not they know it
   c. The other party needs me more than I need them, and I will be sure to make that clear to them

---

2   This test, written by Ellen J Belzer, is based on a case entitled "_Hard/Soft Negotiation Choice_" developed by William Ury, Roger Fisher, and Bruce Patton of the Harvard Program on Negotiation.

_____ 5 **I am usually:**
   a. Hard on the people and hard on the problem
   b. Soft on the people and hard on the problem
   c. Soft on the people and soft on the problem

_____ 6 **When negotiating with another party for the first time, my primary concern is:**
   a. Building a relationship at the same time I am working on the deal (both are necessary at the first meeting)
   b. Building a foundation for a positive future relationship (a deal would be a nice bonus, but the relationship should take precedence during the first meeting)
   c. Getting the deal that brought us to the negotiation in the first place (a relationship would be nice, but the business-at-hand must be the priority)

_____ 7 **My usual style in a negotiation is to:**
   a. Obtain as many concessions as I can from the other party in order to establish control of our relationship
   b. Make concessions to the other party whenever possible in order to demonstrate that I am serious about our relationship
   c. Avoid making concessions that are tied to our relationship

_____ 8 **When I'm involved in a conflict with another party during the negotiation, I am usually the person who:**
   a. Emphasizes the areas of agreement so that we can build on the positive
   b. Emphasizes the problem so that we can address it head-on
   c. Emphasizes both the areas of agreement and the problem so that we don't lose sight of either

_____ 9 **If the other party says something that is just plain wrong or really stupid during a negotiation, I probably would:**
   a. Try to understand their feelings and help them "save face"
   b. Point out their mistake and kindly explain why they're wrong
   c. Change the subject and pretend like I didn't hear it

_____ 10 **Those who know me well probably would describe my communication style (in professional situations) as mainly:**
   a. Forceful, serious, deliberate
   b. Easy going, agreeable, amiable
   c. Direct, objective, open

_____ **11** **When the other party and I are debating a point during the negotiation, I mainly tend to:**
  a. Ask a lot of questions to figure out what the other party finds objectionable
  b. Get the other party to understand my views
  c. Adjust my position to avoid unnecessary conflict

_____ **12** **If I were being filmed during a negotiation, I would most often be seen:**
  a. Making offers
  b. Identifying needs
  c. Making threats

_____ **13** **If I'm selling something, and I know in advance the lowest price for which I'd settle, I would be most likely to:**
  a. Start out by giving the other party a bottom line that is somewhat higher than my real one, in order to test the water and see if I can get more from the deal
  b. Disclose my real bottom line up front, in order to be honest and avoid game-playing
  c. Suggest a range for a possible settlement to see if we're in the same ballpark

_____ **14** **In particularly difficult negotiations, I tend to:**
  a. Accept occasional losses on some of my less important points to avoid spending unnecessary time and energy on debates
  b. Spend more time and energy looking for options that will enable both parties to achieve gains on major points
  c. Insist on gaining my points, while letting others take care of themselves

_____ **15** **For me, the most important determinant of success in a negotiation is:**
  a. Whether the other party was as pleased as I was with the outcome
  b. Whether we've reached a satisfactory agreement
  c. Whether I've achieved all or most of what I came to accomplish

Negotiation self-test

Score Sheet

	Soft	Hard	Principled
1	a	b	c
2	c	a	b
3	b	c	a
4	c	a	b
5	a	c	b
6	c	b	a
7	a	b	c
8	b	a	c
9	b	c	a
10	a	b	c
11	b	c	a
12	c	a	b
13	a	b	c
14	c	a	b
15	c	b	a

Training Tool #38

Ways to frame an
issue in order to get
the desired results

Framing issues

TYPE: Practice exercise

ESTIMATED TRAINING TIME: 45 minutes

THEME: Negotiation

OBJECTIVE:

➡ to understand the difference between distributive and integrative negotiation and
how to frame issues for each type.

MATERIALS NEEDED: A copy of the case study on "Framing Issues" for all participants

PROCEDURE:

In a mini-lecture, describe the differences between distributive negotiation (a fixed-pie
negotiation in which parties decide how to divide the pie) and integrative negotiation (in
which you do not assume a fixed pie and try to identify ways to make the pie bigger).

Next, explain the concept of framing: the words and phraseology used to present the
issue at the negotiating table. Point out that the way in which a question is asked will lead
to a distributive or integrative outcome.

To seek a distributive outcome, focus on the issue and ask a close-ended question that
includes a possible solution. For example: "Should we go to Tampa or San Francisco for
our next educational retreat?" The two possibilities are Tampa and San Francisco; negotiators will most likely decide on one or the other, simply because of the way the question
was phrased.

An integrative negotiation makes it possible to expand the pie by allowing for more
possibilities. Frame these as open-ended questions that get to the larger, underlying question, but do not include possible solutions. (In the example about meeting locations, you
would not mention the cities being considered since those are possible solutions that will
lead to a yes/no response.) It helps to start these questions with the words, "How can
we . . ." For example, "How can we attract the most participants to our educational retreat
by our choice of location?" The outcomes may include Tampa and San Francisco, but
also may include numerous other cities that are affordable, convenient for attendees, and
desirable to visit.

After distributing the instruction sheet, ask participants to divide into small groups of
5–7 people. Ask each group to practice the art of framing by developing a question for this
case in two ways: one that is most likely to lead to a distributive (yes/no) outcome, and

the other that is most likely to result in an integrative (expanded pie) outcome. Give them 20 minutes for their small-group discussions.

DEBRIEFING:

While there may be variations on the wording, an example of distributive framing for this exercise would be: "Should our practice purchase the new x-ray by CYR Bodies, Inc.?" With the question framed in this manner, the practice will decide to buy the new machine or not.

An example of integrative framing would be: "How can we acquire the best possible deal on digital x-ray equipment for our practice at the most reasonable cost?" With this framing, the negotiators may decide to purchase the machine offered by CYR Bodies, Inc., or they may decide on products by other vendors. The integrative question also may result in other outcomes, e.g. leasing a machine, sharing a machine with other practices in the medical office building, etc.

If time permits, ask the following questions:

1   In what types of instances would it be preferable to frame a question as distributive rather than integrative? When would it be best to frame a question as integrative?

2   Was it difficult or easy to formulate these questions? Explain your response.

3   Do you believe that the way an issue is framed has a bearing on the outcome? Why or why not?

4   What impact will knowing these strategies have on your future negotiations? On other types of meetings?

PRACTICE EXERCISE: FRAMING ISSUES

You are about to develop the agenda for the next management staff meeting at your practice, and one of the issues that you will decide concerns the need for a new digital x-ray machine. The cost is an issue, but having a quality machine on-site is very important and the old x-ray is woefully out-of-date.

▶ **Distributive framing:** You have explored several bids, and the one that looks best to you is from CYR Bodies, Inc. You want to make this decision as soon as possible, and decide that it's enough that you have reviewed five other proposals and have selected this company's proposal to present to the group. As such, you have decided to frame the issue in a way that is most likely to result in a distributive outcome, as follows:

▶ **Integrative framing:** Although you have received a reasonably good bid from CYR Bodies, Inc. for a new digital x-ray, you believe that since this is a major expenditure the management staff should consider all of its options carefully. After all, you've received another good offer from Kal-El Digital Systems, and you also wonder what other possibilities might emerge by having all of the managers weigh in. You have decided to ask the question in a way that is most likely to result in an integrative outcome, as follows:

Training Tool #39

The family medicine/managed care contract dilemma

TYPE: Case study

ESTIMATED TRAINING TIME: 30 minutes

THEMES: Negotiation, conflict management, difficult colleagues

OBJECTIVES:
- to understand the importance of reviewing and interpreting all provisions before contracts are negotiated and signed;
- to identify strategies for negotiating multi-party contractual conflicts.

MATERIALS NEEDED: A copy of the case study for all participants

PROCEDURE:
Tell participants that after they have read the case study, they will be asked to discuss the issues involved in this negotiation and how it could be resolved.

DEBRIEFING:
1   What are the major issues involved in this contract dispute?
2   Was it advisable for the family physicians to have threatened a lawsuit?
3   What can be done to reconcile the differences in the parties' perspectives of the other?
4   What can be done to de-escalate the tension?
5   What should both parties do to resolve this situation?
6   What is likely to happen if this dispute is not resolved?
7   What are the major lessons about contracting for physicians from this case study?
8   What are the major lessons for managed care organizations?

CASE STUDY: THE FAMILY MEDICINE/MANAGED CARE CONTRACT DILEMMA

Northwest IPA (composed of 44 family physicians) and Harbortown Managed Care Organization (MCO) are about to renegotiate their contract. These parties have enjoyed a successful relationship for the past 12 years, and the plan covers 40% of the family physicians' patients. Unfortunately, the relationship has soured during the past year, and a major conflict is now threatening to destroy their long-term relationship.

In each of their previous contracts, the family physicians had agreed to different risk pool arrangements in addition to a capitation agreement for primary care services. When the risk pool arrangements weren't working well, the MCO started pressuring the family physicians to decrease utilization. From the MCO's perspective, this was essential to the plan's survival.

From the family physicians' perspective, the MCO had become too fixated on the bottom line and was not appreciative enough of the family physicians' quality performance. They were also upset that the MCO had retroactively corrected a mistake in their data and asked the family physicians to pay back a rather large sum of money to the plan.

Although the family physicians agreed to repay this money, they began to mistrust the MCO and hired an auditor to check the MCO's data. Although the data were found to be accurate, the auditors pointed out that the following phrase in the contract regarding "incentive pool" payments was subject to interpretation:

> "At the end of the period to be reconciled, actual payment for services expensed to each of the Incentive Funds, allowed amount less the stop loss amount (referred to hereafter as adjusted payment), shall be deducted from the total dollars allocated to the Incentive Fund."

As the auditors noted (and the family physicians' attorneys agreed), most of the terms were not defined in the contract. The term "actual payment for services" was the clause in question. The MCO had interpreted "actual payment" to refer to the amount actually paid for services rendered, plus co-pays. As the auditors pointed out, if this term was interpreted as meaning the amount actually paid for services rendered (not including co-pays), the family physicians would be owed a total of $224 704!

Prior to the renegotiation of their contract, the family physicians sent their contracting team to meet with MCO representatives to ask that the MCO pay the family physicians the $224 704. The MCO refused, noting that this provision had never been interpreted any other way throughout its history. The family physicians, bolstered by hearing that they had a strong case, threatened to sue – even though they expected to continue their contract with the plan. The MCO said they would not settle; they would fight the family physicians in court on the basis of principle. They also threatened to "leave the county," i.e. discontinue their contract with the family physicians.

Let's renegotiate

TYPE: Case study

ESTIMATED TRAINING TIME: 30 minutes

THEMES: Negotiation, conflict management

OBJECTIVES:

➡ to understand the importance of fact-finding and identifying one another's expectations;

➡ to discuss the effects of requests for mid-contract renegotiations;

➡ to identify strategies for negotiating contractual conflicts.

MATERIALS NEEDED: A copy of the case study on the following page for all participants

PROCEDURE:

Tell participants that after they have read the case study they will be asked to discuss the issues involved in this negotiation and how it could be resolved.

DEBRIEFING:

1　Is Dr. Deal standing on firm ground by asking for the contract to be renegotiated while the contract is still in force? Why or why not?

2　What could Dr. Deal have done to have avoided this dispute?

3　To what extent, if any, is Mr. Pennywise responsible for the conflict with Dr. Deal?

4　Is there anything that Mr. Pennywise can do to resolve the conflict with Dr. Deal without capitulating to her demands? If so, what?

5　What should Dr. Deal do differently in order to create better possibilities for her future at Littletown Community Health Center? What should Mr. Pennywise do?

CASE STUDY: LET'S RENEGOTIATE

Dr. Sasha Deal has her choice of three practice sites in small rural areas within the State in order to fill a National Health Service Corps (NHSC) obligation. Dr. Deal is only interested in one of the sites (the Littletown Community Health Center) because she heard it was a particularly nice community; she wasn't nearly as impressed with what she'd heard about the other two.

Even though Dr. Deal is repaying her NHSC scholarship obligation, the NHSC tries to give physicians at least some choice of underserved areas when it can, and then each clinic can decide how much it will pay its physicians.

Recently, Dr. Deal sat down with the administrator of the Littletown Community Health Center to negotiate the terms of a potential contract. The administrator, Mr. Perry Pennywise, started out the session by telling Dr. Deal that he was willing to offer $85 000 per year. After hearing about the clinic's many financial problems, Dr. Deal agreed to this amount. The contract was for one year.

After three months, Dr. Deal realized that she was on call a lot more than she had anticipated. She also didn't realize that she'd be spending so much time providing care to all of the community's nursing home patients on a regular basis, including emergencies. But what really got to her was when she heard that the other NHSC doctor in the community who sees fewer patients has a higher salary than she does. Mr. Pennywise defends that, believing that the other physician deserves more as a reward for staying in the community for several years.

Feeling disrespected and under-compensated, Dr. Deal asks for a renegotiation of her contract. Mr. Pennywise refuses, noting that the contract is for a one-year period. Dr. Deal becomes extremely angry, and is bad-mouthing the practice to anyone who will listen. Now she does only what is required of her and no more. While she is currently making plans to leave the area after her contract expires, she will consider staying in the community if Mr. Pennywise comes back with a better offer and particularly if he offers something to make up for what she has been going through.

My way or the highway

TYPE: Case study

ESTIMATED TRAINING TIME: 30 minutes

THEMES: Negotiation, difficult colleagues

OBJECTIVE:

➡ to distinguish between strategies that are most likely to work in one's favor in a negotiation from those that would be disadvantageous.

MATERIALS NEEDED: A copy of the case study on the following page for all participants; a flip chart is optional.

PROCEDURE:

Tell participants that after they have read the case study, they will be asked to identify which of the physician's behaviors would not be recommended for an effective negotiation.

DEBRIEFING:

1 What negotiation gaffes were made in this case? (Write responses on the flip chart and point out which responses refer to communication issues and which refer to the substance and process of the negotiation.)
2 How did Dr. Crank's assumptions about hospital leaders and the process of negotiation affect this interaction?
3 Were all the errors made by Dr. Crank, or were others responsible as well?
4 Was Dr. Crank justified in announcing his bottom line right away? Why or why not? What would be the benefits of engaging in the "dance" of negotiation?
5 How would this negotiation be likely to conclude? What strategies, if any, could have had an impact on Dr. Crank's behavior?
6 What could Dr. Crank have done differently to have achieved his asking price, or close to it?

CASE STUDY: MY WAY OR THE HIGHWAY

At 2:00 pm, the Chief Financial Officer (CFO) and a Vice President of Random Hospital planned to meet with a local physician, Dr. Frasier Crank, to negotiate the terms of selling Dr. Crank's medical practice to the hospital. Dr. Crank has asked for a purchase price of $800 000. Dr. Crank said he would bring his two partners, Drs. Martin and Niles.

The CFO, Roz Boyle, arrived in the conference room early to ensure that copies of the current version of the proposal were neatly placed at each seat around the table. She was joined by Daphne Starr, Vice President for Development. Drs. Martin and Niles arrived at around 2:15 pm, but Ms. Boyle noted that she did not want to start the meeting until Dr. Crank arrived. At 2:40 pm, just as the meeting was about to be canceled, Dr. Crank arrived.

"All right, let's get this over with," Dr. Crank said testily. "I've got a lot to do."

"First, we'd like to welcome you to Random Hospital," Ms. Boyle said.

"Thanks," said Dr. Crank. "Are you going to pay the $800 000 or not?"

Ms. Starr smiled in an effort to establish rapport. "It's nice to see you again, Dr. Crank. I'm sure that today we'll be able to arrive at an equitable price for your practice."

"I know how you people are," Dr. Crank said, "so don't try to pull any fast ones on me. I've had the practice appraised, and we're not taking a penny less than $800 000."

Ms. Starr and Ms. Boyle caught a glimpse of each other, both trying to remain calm. "Dr. Crank, we've seen the appraisal report, and we agree that the building, equipment, aged accounts receivable and other hard assets are definitely worth $700 000. But you are also asking for an additional $100 000 for patient loyalty and the worth of the practice's future value. We consider those to be 'blue sky' items, and we're having a little problem with that."

Dr. Crank stood up and began pacing around the table with his arms folded. "You think patient loyalty and the practice's value are 'blue sky' issues?" Dr. Crank said. "Why am I not surprised? Let me tell you a thing or two. I don't do stupid negotiation games. I've given you our bottom line, now take it or leave it."

"We were hoping for a bit more flexibility on your part, Dr. Crank," Ms. Boyle said. "Dr. Nile, Dr. Martin, do you agree with . . ."

"Well, I think that . . ." Dr. Nile began.

"I speak for all of us," Dr. Crank interjected. "We should even add an extra $100 000 for the aggravation of closing this deal."

Drs. Niles and Martin looked blankly at their partner.

"We've prepared some documents for you," said Ms. Starr. "What we'd like to suggest is . . ."

"Are we wasting our time here?" Dr. Crank interrupted, standing over Ms. Starr. Pointing his finger at Ms. Boyle, he began to raise his voice. "I've asked you a direct question. Are you going to pay our asking price or not?"

"If you're not willing to discuss this issue, we'll have to say no," Ms. Boyle said. "But I think that you . . ."

Dr. Crank grabbed his briefcase and pulled out his car keys. "You people don't know the first thing about me, do you? You probably don't know that I've been responsible for more patient admissions over the last 20 years than most people on your medical staff. You have no clue what I've done for this community."

"We're well aware . . ."

"Last chance," Dr. Crank said. "We're here to make a deal, not to be haggling over nonsense. We've offered you the fair market value of our practice. You said you were interested. Now put your money where your mouth is, or don't waste my time."

Dispute about the
placement of names
on a co-authored
article

Training Tool #42

The squabbling doctors

TYPE: Role play – a recent residency graduate and a well-known physician[3]

(Note: You can alter this exercise by changing the roles to nurse and physician or social worker and administrator, whatever configuration you'd like. For the best results, have the person in the Apple role be the youngest and least experienced of the two.)

ESTIMATED TRAINING TIME: 30 minutes

THEMES: Negotiation, conflict management

OBJECTIVES:

➡ to identify effective ways to negotiate what appears to be a distributive (i.e. fixed pie) negotiation;

➡ to demonstrate the importance of framing the issue in a way that will be most likely to lead to an integrative (make-the-pie-bigger) outcome;

➡ to show that one's ability to negotiate effectively is often dependent on one's ability to accurately discern the differences between each party's real needs;

➡ to show how power differentials can affect the process and outcome.

MATERIALS NEEDED: Copies of the role play exercise for each participant; flip chart is optional

PROCEDURE:

Ask all participants to select a partner. If there are an uneven number of participants, ask the extra person to serve as observer or double up on a role with one of the others. Assign each individual to play an opposing role, perhaps by asking the youngest of the dyad to play the role of Dr. Apple. Announce that everyone will have 15 minutes to negotiate a mutual gains (win-win) solution.

---

3 This role-play exercise is based on the concept of a case that originally appeared in *Dispute Resolution* by Stephen B Goldberg, Eric D Green, and Frank A E Sander (Boston, Little, Brown and Co, 1984), and was later adapted into another version that appeared in the *Negotiation Journal*, April 1990, in an article entitled, "Negotiation Problems and Possible Solutions." Another article by Stephen B Goldberg that addresses this general scenario appeared in the October 1990 issue of *The Negotiation Journal* entitled "The Case of the Squabbling Authors: A 'Med-Arb' Response."

DEBRIEFING:

1 Ask for a show of hands: How many achieved a win-win solution? Were any deadlocked? If so, how did this happen?

2 Ask each dyad to report on their outcomes. (If using a flip chart, jot down the solutions.)

3 What was the specific question that you were negotiating? In other words, how was the conflict "framed," (i.e. defined)?

4 What issues were involved in this dispute?

5 What criteria were used for reaching a decision?

6 What strategies were most effective?

7 Did the solutions meet the real needs of each party?

NOTE TO INSTRUCTORS

The most common way that the issue is framed in this exercise is "whose name should go first?" Point out that this manner of framing the question will result in a win-lose outcome. That is, either Dr. Apple or Dr. Berry will win (getting his/her name first on the byline) while the other will lose (being named second).

On its face, it seems that this role play is about a distributive negotiation – a fixed pie situation that often results in a win-lose outcome. But it doesn't have to be that way! By framing the issue in a way that focuses on the underlying question rather than a question that evokes an either/or response, it is possible to create more opportunities for mutual-gains outcomes.

To consider the underlying question, consider how each party's needs are different. (Point out that in negotiation, even when it seems like both parties want exactly the same thing, there is usually a subtle difference in their needs.) In this case, both Drs. Apple and Berry want credit for their contributions to the article, but the difference is that Dr. Apple wants credit for the work and Dr. Berry wants credit for the idea.

By understanding these different sets of needs, it is then possible to frame the question by asking the underlying question. Rather than "whose name should go first?" which would result in a win-lose outcome, ask, "How can we both obtain appropriate recognition for our respective roles in this project?" This opens the door to a plethora of additional solutions that extend far beyond having one's name first on the byline.

Solutions that are frequently offered for this case are:

➡ **Give Dr. Apple the first position on the byline.** That way, Dr. Apple will be able to advance his/her career by becoming better known. After all, the person whose name appears first in the byline will be most prominent in the indices for journal articles. Surely, this is not the best solution! What about the fact that this article was Dr. Berry's idea?

➡ **Give Dr. Berry the first position on the byline.** This would only seem fair since the concept for the article was Dr. Berry's idea, right? But what about Dr. Apple, who did six months of work on the article? This is not the best solution either. One party wins, the other loses.

➡ **Consider an alphabetical listing.** This is a mediocre solution, at best. After all, since both negotiators already know which last name would come first alphabetically, the person whose name comes later in the alphabet would simply be making a concession to the other.

➡ **Flip a coin.** Yes, it's impartial and it's definitely a quick-fix – but only one party's needs would be met.

➡ **Write a second article and take turns on whose name appears first.** This is a better solution, but not perfect. The good news is that the parties wouldn't be locking themselves into the assumption that there would only be one article. The imperfect part of this solution is that if the two parties have an acrimonious relationship at this point, why commit to another six months of working together and thus prolonging their unfavorable situation?

➡ **Add a footnote to point out who did the bulk of work and who had the major idea.** This is a much better solution since both parties' needs would be met. Remember: no two parties ever want exactly the same thing! In this exercise, Dr. Apple wanted credit for doing the lion's share of the work, while Dr. Berry wanted credit for the idea. With this solution, both of these needs would be met, regardless of whose name appears first in the byline. But the question still looms: Whose name will go first? The dispute may not be entirely over.

➡ **Give Dr. Berry's name to the major idea; e.g. "The Berry Plan," and let Dr. Apple have first credit on the byline.** This solution more specifically meets the needs of each party. By referring to "The Berry Plan" in the title and throughout the article, Dr. Berry will receive much greater credit for the idea than he/she would in a byline alone. By listing Dr. Apple as first author in the byline, Dr. Apple would be able to prove that he/she did the majority of work on the article and would be listed in author bibliographies, which would help his/her career. What's more, each party would be recognized for what they actually did on the article!

ROLE PLAY: THE SQUABBLING DOCTORS

You and a colleague in the Department of Family Medicine have just completed collaborating on an article that will be submitted to a professional journal for publication. The article, which describes a new (and extremely novel) model for the integrated treatment of depression and hypertension, is expected to have a major impact nationwide. The collaboration had been a fairly smooth one until you started doing the title page. At that time, a strong disagreement developed about which of your names should be listed first on the article.

As you negotiate, consider the following:

- Dr. Apple, a recent residency graduate who has been at the medical center for nearly two years, did the bulk of work on the article. In fact, this article took a substantial amount of Dr. Apple's time during the last six months. Dr. Apple did most of the research as well as most of the writing and re-writing. Dr. Apple is 20 years younger than Dr. Berry. Also, Dr. Apple believes this article is essential in advancing his/her career.

- Dr. Berry has been at the medical center for approximately 20 years and is very well known nationally. Dr. Berry has had several major leadership positions in his/her medical specialty association at the local, state, and national levels, and is a widely published author of journal articles and a frequent speaker at medical meetings throughout the country. Dr. Berry contributed the major idea around which the paper is based. Although Dr. Berry spent only a minimal amount of time editing each version of the article, Dr. Berry helped Dr. Apple by directing him/her to the appropriate research sources. Dr. Berry believes that Dr. Apple could not have written the article without his/her leadership and original thinking.

This matter has to be decided quickly in order to submit the article in time for the publisher's deadline.

Training Tool #43

A new lease on life

TYPE: Role play – pharmacy chain owner and landlord

ESTIMATED TRAINING TIME: 30 minutes

THEME: Negotiation

OBJECTIVES:
➡ to develop skills in bargaining on a multi-issue negotiation;
➡ to understand the concepts of concessions, compromises, and creative solutions.

MATERIALS NEEDED: A copy of the two roles for each dyad; a flip chart is optional.

PROCEDURE:
Describe the concepts of concessions, compromises, creative solutions, and trade-offs. Ask each participant to get a partner and distribute the instruction sheets so that each person in the dyads will play an opposing role. Tell participants that their task is to get the best possible deal for themselves on all three points, and that they will have 15 minutes for their negotiation. After time is up, reconvene the dyads for an all-group discussion.

DEBRIEFING:
1 What were your dyad's solutions to the three negotiating points? (Write responses on the flip chart.)
2 Did you make concessions to the other party on any of the points? Did you compromise? Did you invent creative solutions in which both parties' needs were met?
3 If you made concessions to the other party, why did you see the necessity for doing so?
4 Which solutions were the most advantageous to the landlord? To the pharmacy chain owner? What strategies did these negotiators use?

ROLE PLAY: A NEW LEASE ON LIFE
CONFIDENTIAL INSTRUCTIONS

Pharmacy Chain Owner

You have three successful pharmacies in a large city in the Midwest, and plan to add a fourth store. The most desirable option is to move into an available space (1800 square feet, including 450 feet of storage space) in a strip mall that is close to the center of town and only one block from a major medical office building. The space was previously occupied by another pharmacy, but the owner passed away.

Today, you will meet with the landlord, and will sign the lease – but only if you can agree on these three points:

(a) The number of years of the lease:

You prefer a short-term lease (approximately one to two years) in order to determine whether this is a profitable location.

(b) The price of the lease:

You would like to pay no more than $1000 per month; preferably somewhat less. You think you'll do well in this location based on your projections, but you don't want to pay too much in overhead when this store is just starting out.

(c) The condition of the facility:

You are very pleased with the layout of the pharmacy, but believe there is a need for repainting as well as a new carpet. The paint job isn't in bad shape, but it's the ugliest color of green you've ever seen. And the carpet is disgusting. During a recent walk-through, you almost tripped over some worn spots.

ROLE PLAY: A NEW LEASE ON LIFE
CONFIDENTIAL INSTRUCTIONS

Landlord

The pharmacy chain owner that you will meet with today has three successful pharmacies in a large city in the Midwest, and plans to add a fourth store. You are the landlord of a strip mall that is close to the center of town and only one block from a major medical office building. You have the perfect space for the pharmacy chain owner's store. It is 1800 square feet (including 450 square feet of storage space) and has already been designed as a pharmacy. The previous tenant passed away.

You hope to sign the lease today – but only if you can agree on these three points:

(a) The number of years of the lease:

You would like to have a long-term commitment – preferably for five or ten years – for two reasons. First, having a long-term lease would keep you from the hassle of finding a new tenant or having to renegotiate the terms from year to year. Second, although you haven't said this to the pharmacy chain owner, you may decide to sell the building during the next few years, and a long-term lease would be a good selling point.

(b) The price of the lease:

You realize it might be a little high for the Midwest, but you'd like to get $1500 per month for this space – preferably $1750. After all, the location is great for a pharmacy as it's just one block from a major medical building. You're only charging $1000 per month to other tenants in the building, but you think the pharmacy should be worth more because you spent considerable capital having it designed as a pharmacy. You don't think the pharmacy owner knows what other tenants in the mall are paying.

(c) The condition of the facility:

In order to save money, you'd prefer to rent the space "as is." While you realize that the carpeting has gotten pretty worn, you don't think it's that bad. You had the space painted only two years ago in your favorite shade of green. In any event, you really don't want to shell out any more capital on this space than you already have.

A salary negotiation

TYPE: Role play – physician and administrator

ESTIMATED TRAINING TIME: 60 minutes

THEME: Negotiation

OBJECTIVES:

➡ to demonstrate the importance of identifying goals, target point, reservation point, and starting point in advance of negotiations that involve bargaining;

➡ to identify bargaining strategies that result in fair, win-win outcomes.

MATERIALS NEEDED: A copy of the two roles for each dyad

PROCEDURE:

Ask each participant to select a partner. Distribute the role of "administrator" to one person in each dyad and the role of "physician" to the other. After participants have read their confidential instructions, ask them to spend 8–10 minutes determining their "bargaining zone" by identifying their goal (highest aspiration), reservation point (lowest acceptable offer), target point (where they want or expect to end up), and starting point (opening offer). Tell them to "guesstimate" the same for the other party.

Announce that everyone will have 30 minutes to negotiate a mutual gains (win-win) solution, and to make the best possible deal for themselves or their organization. When time is up, bring participants back together for an all-group discussion.

DEBRIEFING:

1   How many achieved a win-win solution? What were each dyad's outcomes?

2   Did anyone *not* reach agreement on the contract? If so, what happened?

3   How many of those who played the role of physician found out that the administrator could have paid up to $180 000? Knowing this, are they as happy with the results? What does this say about how much to reveal to the other party?

4   Of those who played the role of the family physician, did they disclose what they earned when they were in solo practice? Why or why not?

5   To what extent were the negotiations affected by the statistics regarding starting salaries? How did they deal with the different sets of statistics acquired by the two characters?

6   To what extent did their preparation (determining goals, reservation points, target points and starting points) help them to make a better deal?

7 Did the solutions meet the real needs of each party?

8 How many reached agreement on matters other than the salary? For example, did they also reach agreement on other parts of the package such as work schedule, vacations, CME travel, moving expenses, insurance benefits, professional liability insurance, bonuses, and other aspects of usual employment agreements?

9 If they did reach agreement on other items in addition to salary, how does that affect the value of the entire package?

10 Did they address the issue of working on Saturdays and weeknights? If so, how?

ROLE PLAY: A SALARY NEGOTIATION
CONFIDENTIAL INSTRUCTIONS

Administrator

You are the Administrator of Halenharty Community Health Center (HCHC) and you have been interviewing physicians for the last three weeks to join your staff. Of six applicants, you are most interested in a board-certified family physician with six years experience in private solo practice in a small rural community in your State. You believe that this particular applicant, who has certificates of added qualifications in geriatrics and adolescent medicine, is head and shoulders above any of the other applicants you've interviewed. This physician is also a widely published author of journal articles on various health care delivery topics. You believe he/she would enhance the reputation of HCHC.

The physician is coming in today to negotiate an employment contract. When you met with this physician before, you offered $100 000 (a little higher than the $90 000 that you normally paid as a starting salary for family physicians in the past, but still on the low side of statistics you found showing that starting salaries for family physicians range from $90 000 to $150 000). The physician was noncommittal about both the job and the salary during the first meeting. You do have a reserve fund that you could tap into (you could even pay up to $180 000 if you tap into this fund), but you'd prefer to save as much as you can for the peaks and valleys that HCHC often experiences. HCHC has only recently gotten out-of-the-red and you'd like to keep it that way! The other two family physicians on your staff now earn $135 000 and $160 000 each, but one has been at the center for three years and the other for more than eight years. You know that other health centers pay more, but a large number of your center's patients are indigent and the center simply doesn't have the resources to match what others are offering.

Naturally, your objective is to save as much money as you can, while still getting the physician on your staff. You would like this physician on your staff as soon as possible. Demands on HCHC have been tremendous lately, and staffing problems are most problematic on Saturdays and weeknights. If this physician does not accept your offer, the physician who is your next choice would probably take the position for $100,000, maybe even less, but you'd prefer to hire the physician you are meeting with today.

	YOUR:		**THEIR: (estimated)**
Goal	_____		_____
Reservation point	_____		_____
Target point	_____		_____
Starting point	_____		_____

ROLE PLAY: A SALARY NEGOTIATION
CONFIDENTIAL INSTRUCTIONS

Family Physician

You are a family physician who has been in solo private practice in a rural community in this State for the last six years. You are board-certified and have certificates of added qualifications in geriatrics and adolescent medicine. Plus, you are a widely published author of journal articles on various health care delivery topics.

You were quite happy in your old practice, but as the local economy deteriorated, large numbers of the population moved out of town. When you started your practice there, you made around $90000 per year. However, last year you made $75000. You've been interested in joining the Halenharty Community Health Center (HCHC) because (a) you like the people; (b) you don't want to work in a solo practice anymore and HCHC has two other doctors on staff; and (c) you've heard many good things about HCHC for years.

Today, you are meeting with the administrator of HCHC to negotiate your contract. You've met the administrator once before, and during that meeting you were offered $100000. You said you wanted to think about it. Everything looks fine to you about the contract except that you'd prefer a higher salary – if possible, a *much* higher salary. You recently read statistics from a physician recruitment firm showing that your State's average starting salary for family physicians is $144000 and $149000 for those that include obstetrics. However, you don't know if these figures represent what is paid by community health centers. (You don't plan to include OB in your practice.) Since these figures are the "average," you'd like to get substantially more because, after all, you are highly qualified. You also want to be guaranteed that you will not have to work on Saturdays.

If you don't work out an employment agreement with HCHC, your next best option is to accept a position with a clinic in another area at a starting salary of $126000 with a $4000 raise in six months. However, you're not nearly as impressed with that clinic as you are with HCHC.

YOUR:		THEIR: (estimated)
Goal	_____	_____
Reservation point	_____	_____
Target point	_____	_____
Starting point	_____	_____

Training Tool #45

The contract deadline

TYPE: Role play – physician and administrator

ESTIMATED TRAINING TIME: 60 minutes

THEME: Negotiation

OBJECTIVE:

➡ to explore ways to handle a multi-issue employment dispute in which some of the issues have become personalized.

MATERIALS NEEDED: A copy of the two roles for each dyad

PROCEDURE:

Ask each participant to select a partner. Distribute the role of "administrator" to one person in the dyad and the role of "Dr. Fester" to the other.

Announce that everyone will have 35 minutes to negotiate a mutual gains (win-win) solution, and to make the best possible deal for themselves or the organization.

DEBRIEFING:

1 How did the animosities between the characters affect their ability to come to agreement? How were the ill feelings handled?
2 Did the administrator hurt or help the negotiation by making an ultimatum?
3 Did your characters reach agreement on the employment contract? If so, what terms were agreed to in regard to Dr. Fester's four demands? Was the contract for a one-year period or longer?
4 Which of the four issues was most difficult to agree upon? Why?
5 What strategies did both parties use to come to a successful resolution?
6 If an agreement was not reached, what factors were responsible?

ROLE PLAY: THE CONTRACT DEADLINE
CONFIDENTIAL INSTRUCTIONS

Dr. Fester

You are one of three physicians who works at Clinica de Salud de Centerville, with a patient population mainly consisting of migrant and seasonal farmworkers – and you are thinking of leaving. You are a National Health Service Corps physician and still have two years to go on your service obligation. However, you are thinking of asking for immediate reassignment due to problems with the administrator. In a discussion with the administrator last week, you refused to sign a new contract with the clinic for the next year unless several demands were met. The administrator told you that the lack of a signed contract within 10 days would be considered as your resignation.

You do not trust the administrator and believe that he/she has lied to you in the past. The administrator promised you certain things (such as a year-end bonus) and then did not keep that promise. (The administrator said that the Board of Directors would not authorize it.) You feel that broken promises occur all too often.

You also believe that the administrator interferes in the clinical practice of medicine, especially by questioning things in your charts. On one occasion, the administrator asked why you prescribed a certain drug! Also, while you've been late getting some of your charts done, you don't think that doing the charts within a few days is unreasonable, as busy as you are. Further, you do not believe the administrator is justified in asking you to be on call every second or third night since it interferes with your family life. Sometimes you get to the office late because you've often had emergencies that have kept you up the night before.

You consider your work at the clinic as "just a job" rather than as a permanent career. You feel little sense of commitment to the clinic or to the community. Because your patients are transient, you feel frustrated with your inability to provide continuing and comprehensive care.

You also believe your salary is too low (currently $125 000). So, you have demanded (a) an increase in pay; (b) greater autonomy in medical practice matters; (c) that you not be required to be on call so frequently; and (d) greater professional respect.

Since the deadline is getting near, you will meet with the administrator now.

ROLE PLAY: THE CONTRACT DEADLINE
CONFIDENTIAL INSTRUCTIONS

Administrator

You are the Administrator of Clinicas de Salud de Centerville, with a patient population mainly consisting of migrant and seasonal farm workers, and it is quite upsetting to you that the center is in danger of losing one of its three physicians. Dr. Fester is a National Health Service Corps physician and still has two years to go on his/her service obligation. It seems that Dr. Fester's problem is with you. In a discussion last week, Dr. Fester refused to sign a new contract with the clinic for the next year unless several demands were met. You brushed off those demands and told Dr. Fester that the lack of a signed contract within 10 days would be considered as his/her resignation.

You are not terribly fond of Dr. Fester who you believe has a bad attitude. However, you believe it is best to try to get Dr. Fester to sign on for another year because of your difficulty in recruiting new physicians. You are certain that if Dr. Fester leaves, your other physicians will be even more stressed than they are now.

Although you believe Dr. Fester provides quality care – at least as far as you know – you are concerned that he/she doesn't comply with the clinic's rules. For example, you are concerned that Dr. Fester often comes to work late, causing a number of scheduling problems for frontline staff and your new Family Nurse Practitioner who has to appease the patients while they wait. You are also concerned that Dr. Fester often does not fill out charts on the same day the patient is seen.

You believe it is possible to pay Dr. Fester more than the $125 000 salary he/she is making now (you could go up to $165 000 if necessary), but you don't like the idea of rewarding someone with a bad attitude who does not comply with clinic rules. Also, you need each of your physicians to work two or three nights a week because most of the migrant and seasonal farm workers who utilize the clinic often cannot come into the center during the work day.

It is not clear to you why Dr. Fester does not feel a greater responsibility to the clinic. You've even worried about whether Dr. Fester's attitude has affected the quality of care. Once or twice, you've gone through Dr. Fester's charts to see if you could notice any irregularities because you didn't think the other doctors would tell you if there were any problems. You questioned Dr. Fester about his/her use of a particular drug, and don't understand why he/she got so defensive. You wondered if Dr. Fester was trying to hide something.

Although you feel that a great deal of stress in your job is due to Dr. Fester, some of the stress is because your community Board of Directors doesn't seem to back you up in your decisions. For example, last year you promised all of your physicians a year-end bonus, but the Board decided to use the extra money for a new patient education outreach program and you were not able to keep your word to the physicians. The Board did not back up your decisions on two or three other occasions.

Although you'd like to work things out with Dr. Fester, you've just about had it. In keeping with your ultimatum to "sign or resign," you need Dr. Fester to sign the contract soon because the 10-day deadline is almost up. Your meeting with Dr. Fester is about to begin.

Training Tool #46

An interagency agreement

TYPE: Role play – State health agency, tax-supported clinic, and community health center

ESTIMATED TRAINING TIME: 90 minutes

THEMES: Negotiation, conflict management

OBJECTIVES:

➠ to show the importance of weighing pros and cons in any type of decision;

➠ to explore solutions that would best meet a specific community's health care needs.

MATERIALS NEEDED: A copy of General Instructions for all participants and a copy of the three roles for each triad

PROCEDURE:

Divide participants into groups of three. Distribute the General Instructions to everyone and then give one of the three roles to persons in each triad so that they are each playing a different role. Point out that the negotiation should be completed within 35 minutes. When time is up, conduct an all-group discussion.

DEBRIEFING:

1   Did your group give the contract to HCHC or to PCS? Or was some other agreement reached? Explain the rationale for your decision.

2   Was the Division justified in reconsidering the contract after the deadline? Why or why not?

3   What amount did the Division agree to give to the entity they selected?

4   What value did HCHC and PCS bring to the table? Did it matter whether PCS was concerned for its survival? Why or why not?

5   How did the Division weigh the pros and cons of selecting either PCS or HCHC? To what extent were factors such as staffing, services, community needs, and proximity taken into account?

6   What were the Division of Family Health's major needs and interests? How did their needs and interests differ from those of the other two parties?

ROLE PLAY: AN INTERAGENCY AGREEMENT

General Instructions

The Division of Family Health is administering a program to provide insurance coverage for prenatal care and delivery for uninsured pregnant women in the State. The program was initiated by the State Legislature in response to the Governor's pledge to do something about the State's extremely high infant mortality rates. In general, the program was designed to assure quality, comprehensive care to uninsured women, including nutrition, mental health services, and health education.

The Division of Family Health is particularly committed to improving prenatal care in the southeastern part of the State, which has a particularly high concentration of uninsured women. Because of the hilly terrain, this area is often referred to as "the Dunes." The Dunes has a population of 3500 people and a drawing population of 3000 more. Many of the women who reside in the Dunes have never had prenatal care before.

Primary Care Services Inc. (PCS) is located in the very heart of the Dunes. Created five years ago, PCS is a federally qualified tax-supported clinic, which provides care to patients throughout the Dunes on a sliding-scale basis. Until this year, the clinic's financial situation has been precarious at best. PCS is staffed by a physician assistant who comes in five days a week, and two family physicians that come in once a week each from Southtown, which is about 50 miles from the Dunes. One of the family physicians has obstetrical privileges at the Southtown Community Hospital; the other does some gynecological procedures, but no obstetrics.

Harrington Community Health Center (HCHC) is a large community health center located about 10 miles from the Southtown Hospital and 60 miles from the Dunes. About 20% of HCHC's patients drive in from the Dunes. HCHC is a full-service clinic with three full-time family physicians (two of whom do deliveries), one obstetrician, two physician assistants, and one nurse practitioner. All of the physicians at HCHC have privileges at Southtown Hospital.

The Division of Family Health was about to enter into a $100 000 contract with HCHC to provide outreach and wrap-around services to uninsured women who reside in the Dunes. However, just before the Division was about to have the papers signed, several angry calls came in from PCS representatives who said they were not informed of the grant. PCS also noted that if HCHC obtains the $100 000 for prenatal outreach and wrap-around services in the Dunes, they will start getting even more of PCS's patients and PCS may not survive. Even worse, they are concerned that their patients who live within the Dunes or in proximity will not have the access to health care that they currently enjoy. Because of the hills in the area and the low-income of community residents, transportation is a major problem. The central location of PCS within the Dunes makes it ideal for those who live in and around the area to obtain their care there.

There has been very little direct communication between PCS and HCHC since word got out about the possible contract with HCHC, but there has been a lot of public name-calling by both entities. At a recent Division staff meeting, it was agreed that the contract was back in play and that a decision would not be made until a meeting could be held to discuss this issue further. That meeting is about to begin.

ROLE PLAY: AN INTERAGENCY AGREEMENT
CONFIDENTIAL INSTRUCTIONS

Division of Family Health

You made an initial decision to contract with HCHC because it obviously has a lot to offer the uninsured pregnant women in the Dunes. PCS didn't even apply for the contract, but their representatives told you recently that they didn't even know about the available funding until it was too late. You are suspicious about this, as you had been told that every possible applicant had been notified.

It was a major decision for you to even agree to this meeting. You thought the decision was a "done deal" to contract with HCHC, but you decided to reconsider when PCS said that they didn't even know the funds were available. While you worry whether it is fair to let PCS get into the process after missing the deadline (which they may or may not have been notified about), you want to do what is best for the uninsured pregnant women in this area. Maybe after today's meeting, you'll know what to do.

Could you have been too hasty to initially select HCHC? Both have their strong points. You have just seen recent statistics showing that pregnant women in the Dunes who have been treated at PCS have better outcomes than those who have visited HCHC. It seems that it should be the other way around, but the data shows otherwise. You wonder why this could be. PCS has been providing the majority of health care services in the Dunes for the last five years. (Until PCS was established, there was no care available in the Dunes' immediate area at all.) You also are aware that patients in the Dunes find it very easy to access PCS, whereas it will be much more difficult for them to visit HCHC. With all the hills and rugged terrain, transportation is a major issue in the Dunes. Maybe that is why most pregnant women who live in the Dunes go to PCS for care.

On the other hand, HCHC really has its act together. They offer many more services, proximity to the hospital, and an outstanding team of providers who are there when people need them. They are superbly qualified to handle the requirements of this project, and their proposal could be a model for others to emulate.

You are open to any workable solution to this problem. You do have a total grant of $250,000, but there are many needs in other parts of the State as well. The $100 000 grant to one of these entities is more than will be allocated for this project in any other part of the State.

ROLE PLAY: AN INTERAGENCY AGREEMENT
CONFIDENTIAL INSTRUCTIONS

Primary Care Services Inc. (PCS)

You did not apply for this contract with the Division of Family Health originally because nobody at PCS knew about it. Actually, your clinic administrator did find the Division's notice about the prenatal initiative on his desk a few weeks ago, but by the time he found it, it was too late.

After you got word that HCHC would get the contract, your Board of Directors (who are publicly elected) got very upset. HCHC already sees about 20% of the patients who reside in the Dunes, and it would be very damaging to PCS if more patients are lost to HCHC. Until this year, PCS was still in the red; currently, they are barely making ends meet.

In regard to quality of care at PCS, you admit that there have been inconsistencies in some areas, but your providers do a wonderful job of treating pregnant women. In fact, a recent study shows that patient outcomes for pregnancy care are superior to those provided by other health centers in the region – and that includes HCHC! The physician assistant that provides care at PCS five days a week not only provides excellent care, but is beloved throughout the community. The same can be said for the two physicians who come to PCS once a week.

You believe that PCS should be given the contract for several reasons: PCS is located right in the middle of the Dunes; most pregnant women in and around the area come to PCS (perhaps due to the transportation issues); you have surprisingly great outcomes for pregnancy care; and your providers know the local people a lot better than HCHC which is 60 miles away. In addition, you do not like the idea of "outsiders" coming in when your clinic can handle this project on its own.

In addition to getting this contract, you hope that you can convince the Division of Family Health Services to give PCS $175 000 rather than the $100 000 that they have designated for this area. You have heard that the Division has a total grant of $250 000 to draw from. With $175,000, you can even try to recruit a full-time family physician with obstetrical privileges as well as one or two family nurse practitioners. (You do not believe that the Dunes could attract a full-time OB, however.)

Above all, you do not want your clinic to fold, which you believe is likely to happen if HCHC takes even 15% of PCS's existing patients. You believe that HCHC is "empire building" at your expense, and many staff members of PCS have been very vocal about that publicly.

ROLE PLAY: AN INTERAGENCY AGREEMENT
CONFIDENTIAL INSTRUCTIONS

Harrington Community Health Center (HCHC)

You do not like the idea that the funding for this contract is being held up because the people from PCS are complaining. They could have applied for the contract but they didn't. Besides, you believe that HCHC provides a much more complete array of services than PCS and is far better qualified to fulfill the needs of this project. You simply want the Division of Family Health to give you the funding as planned so that you can get this project underway. You cannot figure out why the Division is even allowing PCS to enter this discussion after missing the deadline.

In your opinion, there is no contest between HCHC and PCS. While PCS has a physician assistant providing care five days a week and two physicians who visit once a week, HCHC is a full-service clinic with three full-time family physicians (two of whom do deliveries), one obstetrician, two physician assistants, and one nurse practitioner. All of the physicians at HCHC have privileges at Southtown Hospital. Even if PCS gets the contract, there is no way that PCS can offer the range of services that your outstanding team currently provides.

What you haven't yet revealed is that your large community health center (with a community Board of Directors) is now trying to get larger. You have been trying to expand your services into the Dunes for a long time, and this seems to be the perfect opportunity to get your foot in the door. When this project begins, you plan to start by rotating in providers who could be located at a site on the west side of the Dunes that can be used as a temporary clinic until this project is completed. After that, there has been some discussion within your Board of Directors about possibly putting in a permanent satellite clinic in the Dunes someday. This project would help to give you a better assessment about whether that would be feasible.

The $100 000 will be great (you didn't expect that this much would be available), and you hope the Division will let you know today that they've decided on HCHC so you can get started. You're tired of the PCS people whining about losing patients, staying in business, and all of that. People won't be without services when HCHC comes to town.

| **Training Tool #47** |

Hot topic

TYPE: Role play:
➡ City Council
➡ Local Medical Society
➡ Public Health Agency
➡ Restaurant Association
➡ Rights for Business Owners Organization
➡ Tobacco Industry Association

ESTIMATED TRAINING TIME: 90 minutes

THEMES: Negotiation, conflict management

OBJECTIVE:
➡ to understand the complexities of a multi-party negotiation involving a hotly contested public health issue.

MATERIALS NEEDED: A copy of the General Instructions for all participants and a copy of a different character role for persons in each small group

PROCEDURE:
Break into groups of six persons each. Distribute a copy of the General Instructions to all participants, and give a different character role to each player in the small groups. If there is an uneven number of players, double up the roles or assign extras to serve as observers. Note that participants will have 45–60 minutes to negotiate this case.

DEBRIEFING:
1 Was it possible to reach consensus within the time limit for this exercise? Why or why not? If your group didn't reach consensus, was that the direction the negotiation was going?
2 What are the specific issues involved in this dispute?
3 What, if any, are the common interests among the parties? What were the areas of agreement (e.g. did all parties agree about the harmful effects of smoking)?
4 If you played a role that did not support your own views, what did you learn about negotiation by seeing this case through another's eyes?
5 Did any of the parties align with others? If so, which? Why?
6 Did your group address the medical society's suggestion for additional anti-smoking measures? If not, why not? If so, what actions were taken?

7 What did your group do to create effective group dynamics and reduce tensions? How well were difficult behaviors handled? Were efforts made to help those "acting out" to save face?

8 Did your group address how parties felt about the government's role in protecting public health? About whether public health supersedes the right of businesses and customers to choose? If so, what were the agreements and/or sticking points?

9 Did the manner in which issues were framed have an impact on the outcome?

10 What strategies were used for conducting the negotiation and reaching consensus among persons/groups with such disparate and strongly held views?

11 What were the results of your negotiation? What creative solutions did your group develop, if any?

12 What did you learn most from this exercise about negotiating a hotly contested topic?

ROLE PLAY: HOT TOPIC
GENERAL INSTRUCTIONS

Proposal

The City Council has proposed an ordinance to ban indoor smoking in all public spaces. No such ordinance has been adopted in the City as of yet, especially since tobacco companies have a major presence in this area and have been a major source of tax revenues.

As proposed, the ordinance would ban smoking in all workplaces, bars, and restaurants. Smoking would be allowed only in private homes, private residences, and private motor vehicles unless used for child care or day care. Smoking also would be allowed in non-enclosed areas of public places such as restaurant patios and parks.

The History

Recent statistics show that 20.9% of the city's population smoke cigarettes, pipes, or cigars. Nearly half of the surrounding municipalities already have smoking bans, so the City Council decided it was time to propose a ban here as well.

The Council knew there would be extensive public debate on this issue, but didn't realize that this topic would be front page news in the *Daily Gazette* every day for the weeks since the ordinance was introduced. The debate has been unusually polarizing; people on each side of this issue feel quite strongly about their positions and seem to have little tolerance for other views.

The City Council will not decide this issue until an effort has been made to get as much consensus as possible from several groups with an interest in this matter. Those who will attend today's meeting include representatives from:
▶ City Council
▶ Local Medical Society
▶ Public Health Agency
▶ Restaurant Association
▶ Rights for Business Owners Organization
▶ Tobacco Industry Association

ROLE PLAY: HOT TOPIC
CONFIDENTIAL INSTRUCTIONS

Member of the City Council

Most members of the Council support the ban because most are nonsmokers them-selves and would prefer to live in a clean, healthy city. They knew there would be opposition to the proposal, but were surprised to be so deluged by emails, letters, and phone calls from constituents that do not favor this ban. Restaurant and bar owners, various business rights organizations, and representatives of the area's tobacco industry (one of the largest employer groups in the state) have been among the major protestors, as well as members of the public who feel that they should have the right to choose. To give these persons an opportunity to air their views, the Council has called for this meeting to identify areas in which agreement might be possible.

Because the City Council called this meeting, you will lead the discussion. While you will try to be open and objective in order to hear all views, you will also represent the Council's position in support of a smoking ban, which is based on the following:

- ▶ Recent studies acquired by the Council show that most bars and restaurants do not lose substantial business by establishing a smoking ban.

- ▶ A smoking ban in the City will probably not adversely affect tobacco companies in the area because the demand for tobacco products is still quite prevalent nationwide and around the world. It may even be possible for the City to attract new jobs into the area as a result of a smoking ban; several nearby communities have reported that jobs in their areas have increased since smoking bans were adopted.

- ▶ The majority of studies on the effects of smoking bans support the claim that there is no negative economic impact on local businesses. (However, studies show that there have been notable drops in tourism, and that is a major concern to you.)

- ▶ A recent survey of local residents shows that 60% favor a smoking ban in ALL public places.

As a member of City Council, you want to convince the group that adopting the citywide ban is in the best interests of everyone's health, and that this is the way the country is headed.

ROLE PLAY: HOT TOPIC
CONFIDENTIAL INSTRUCTIONS

Member of the Restaurant Association

The majority of your members do NOT want this ban – and that will be the position you will take at this meeting. Your association represents most of the city's restaurants as well as bars and taverns that offer food services. The positions you will argue at today's meeting include the following:

▶ Many restaurant owners are concerned that patrons will stand outside to smoke, thus holding up table turnover.

▶ If smoking is not allowed in designated areas of restaurants and bars, you believe that patrons will go to outlying communities where smoking is still allowed.

▶ You and other restaurant owners are not convinced about the validity of studies showing that business either stays the same or improves when smoking bans are adopted. You believe that your members are in much closer touch with customers than other groups represented at this meeting, and your internal surveys show that an overwhelming number of smokers who frequent these restaurants and bars plan to eat at home more if the ban is enacted.

▶ You believe that it should be the right of business owners to decide whether to allow smoking. Tobacco is, after all, a legal substance.

▶ You know many restaurant owners that have invested heavily in clean-air purifying devices and ventilation systems for their smoking rooms. Some have spent many thousands of dollars on this equipment.

▶ You tend to get *very* testy when people seem to imply that you don't care about people's well being. Part of people's well being is the right to make a living. Restaurant business has been down ever since 9/11 and also due to rising gas prices, both of which have caused people to stay home more. You don't want anything else to affect the livelihood of your members.

▶ If a smoking ban is enacted, you believe that there should be a period of time (maybe a year) over which the ban is phased in. (During that time, you hope to reintroduce another proposed policy that would void the ban.)

You are *very emotional* about this issue. When you get angry, only calm down if someone at the negotiating table says or does something that would make you change your behavior in real life.

ROLE PLAY: HOT TOPIC

CONFIDENTIAL INSTRUCTIONS

Member of the Local Medical Society

The local Medical Society, which you represent, has been among the most vocal supporters of the smoking ban. The society believes this ban is long overdue and that ALL indoor public places should be required to ban smoking. The society also believes that the ban doesn't go far enough. In fact, it proposes two additions to the ordinance:

▶ That smoking must also be banned in outdoor areas that are within a fixed distance of entrances to all public places (including outdoor dining areas, patios, and sidewalks) and also must be banned in city and county recreation facilities such as lakefronts, parks, etc;

▶ That the sale of tobacco products and/or byproducts in retail outlets with store-based clinics must be banned. As the society's president noted during a press conference, "Patients deserve to be kept healthy. Selling any type of tobacco products in any facility that provides health care – including store-based clinics – is absolutely ludicrous."

In support of the smoking ban, the society notes the following:

▶ Approximately 90% of lung cancer deaths and approximately 80–90% of COPD deaths are attributable to smoking.

▶ For every individual who dies from a smoking-related disease, 20 more have a serious illness related to smoking.

▶ The proposed ordinance would protect the public from second-hand smoke, which research shows causes the same health problems as direct smoking: cardiovascular disease, stroke, lung cancer, chronic lung disease, emphysema, bronchitis, and asthma. It is particularly important to protect children, pregnant women, the elderly, and those with health problems from second-hand smoke.

▶ Health care costs are around 40% higher for smokers than nonsmokers.

▶ Smoking bans make it easier for smokers to quit.

You are not moved by arguments about the "rights" of smokers, the "rights" of small business owners, or the "rights" of people to decide on their own whether to visit a smoking establishment. The Medical Society is adamant that the public's health must be paramount.

ROLE PLAY: HOT TOPIC
CONFIDENTIAL INSTRUCTIONS

Member of Local Public Health Agency

On behalf of your agency, you believe a ban on smoking should be implemented immediately for all public places for the following reasons:

▶ There have been numerous studies showing a long list of health improvements for employees, customers, and members of the public-at-large when smoking bans are implemented.

▶ You also have studies showing that business in restaurants and bars in cities that have banned smoking normally goes *up*, not down.

▶ Your agency is concerned with both public health and the environment. In regard to the latter, you oppose any form of pollution.

▶ At some point during this meeting, you will strongly imply that restaurant owners and casino owners do not really care about the health and well-being of their customers – *or* their employees.

▶ You are aware that business owners think there should be designated areas for smokers, but you believe that this is a bogus argument. You have numerous studies showing that second-hand smoke can seep into rooms regardless of air purifiers, filters and other devices. (You do admit that ventilation systems vastly improve air quality, but believe that such systems are not a suitable substitute for a smoking ban.)

▶ Because of accidents caused by people smoking while driving, you believe that smoking also should be banned in all motor vehicles. However, you realize that this will be hard to "sell" at this meeting – and even harder to enforce.

While you strongly support the smoking ban, your agency will be responsible for monitoring and compliance. That is, your employees will have to go to businesses, restaurants, bars and taverns to see if the bans are being upheld and to assess fines or other penalties if they are not. You do not believe that you have enough employees to do this to the degree that will be required, so you will be quite insistent that the City Council provide your agency with additional funds for this extra responsibility. You would like to have around $250 000 for this purpose.

ROLE PLAY: HOT TOPIC
CONFIDENTIAL INSTRUCTIONS

Rights for Business Owners Organization

Your organization is adamant that business owners should have the right to decide for themselves whether to allow smoking in their establishments. Your members believe that this is strictly a business decision – it is not the government's role to police what adults may and may not do! Following is more information about your position:

▶ The position of your organization – which is to allow business owners to decide for themselves whether to allow smoking – is backed by the American Civil Liberties Union.

▶ Your organization believes strongly that free market competition must prevail. In other words, it's up to the public to decide whether or not to give their money to one business over another. Your motto is "Let people vote with their feet." That is, if people do not want to visit a smoking establishment, they can simply take their business elsewhere.

▶ Your organization has a large legal fund for lawsuits that would protect business owners' rights, and your Board of Directors has been strongly considering taking this matter to court if the smoking ban is enacted. On the other hand, the Board may not authorize the funds for this purpose because they don't expect to win the case. (Courts have tended to side with cities and municipalities on this issue, referring to their rights to take measures to protect public safety.) Several members of your Board prefer to use the legal fund for a case that is more likely to win. Still, using the funds for this case remains a possibility.

▶ You believe that health care costs will actually *increase* in the long-term as a result of a smoking ban, because people will live longer.

▶ You believe that restaurants, bars, casinos, and other public venues will experience a great financial hardship if they lose their smoking customers. This will affect the owners, the workers, and even whether the business stays open.

ROLE PLAY: HOT TOPIC
CONFIDENTIAL INSTRUCTIONS

Tobacco Industry Association

Your association represents all of the tobacco processing plants, manufacturers, and warehouses in the area. The tobacco industry is one of the largest employers in the state and you are quite proud of all of the tax revenues from your industry that have contributed to the city's economy.

You are certain that some persons at this meeting will be quite surprised – perhaps shocked – by some of your association's positions, as noted below:

▶ Not surprisingly, your association believes that tobacco should remain a legal substance.

▶ Here's the surprise: although your association won't promote a ban on smoking, it *does not oppose* smoking restrictions in public places such as offices, shopping centers, restaurants, or other unrestricted areas! This is for two reasons: (a) the threat of further restrictions on the tobacco industry if you do not admit to the harmful effects of smoking and second-hand smoke; and (b) your association realizes that some people do prefer to be in smoke-free environments.

▶ While you do not oppose bans in most public places, you believe that reasonable exceptions should be made. For example, you believe that bars, taverns, and other age-restricted facilities should be able to establish their own smoking policies, particularly in places where alcohol is served.

▶ Your association believes that the City Council should take into account that the tobacco industry in the area that you represent has contributed millions of dollars to the local economy and many thousands of jobs – not to mention that members of your association have contributed to the campaigns of several City Council members.

Picture perfect

TYPE: Role play – official from a VA hospital and president of a photography studio

ESTIMATED TRAINING TIME: 30 minutes

THEME: Negotiation

OBJECTIVE:

➡ to identify ethical issues in a negotiated agreement.

MATERIALS NEEDED: A copy of the two roles for each dyad

PROCEDURE:

Ask each participant to select a partner. Distribute one of each role to the parties in each dyad. Announce that everyone will have 15 minutes to negotiate a mutual gains (win-win) solution, and to make the best possible deal for themselves/their organizations.

DEBRIEFING:

1   How many of you reached agreement in this case? What was your end result? Would the pamphlets be distributed or discarded? What dollar amount was agreed upon, if any?
2   For those playing the role of the hospital official, did you tell the studio owner that the photos had already been printed? What ethical issues are involved in not revealing that? When is the omission of information ethical? When is it not?

Point out that a version of this situation actually occurred in real life. As noted in *The Manager as Negotiator: Bargaining for Cooperation and Competitive Gain* by David Lax and James K. Sebenius, Teddy Roosevelt was campaigning for president on a whistle-stop tour and planned to give speeches from the back of the train and distribute a small pamphlet to the citizens who attended. Three million pamphlets had been printed. A campaign worker noticed that there was a small line on the photo that said "Moffett Studios – Chicago." With Moffett holding the copyright, it would cost the campaign $1 per reproduction for unauthorized use – a total of $3 million! Roosevelt's campaign manager, George Perkins, was asked to handle the problem and realized that the campaign didn't have nearly enough money to pay the $3 million fee for the photographs. He sent a cable to Moffitt Studios that said, "We are planning to distribute many pamphlets with Roosevelt's picture on the cover. It will be great publicity for the studio whose photograph we use. How much will you pay us to use yours?" The Moffitt Studio soon wrote back and asked if the campaign would accept $250. They did.

ROLE PLAY: PICTURE PERFECT
CONFIDENTIAL INSTRUCTIONS

Official from VA Hospital

For the last five years you have been an assistant to the commander at the VA Hospital in your area. In May of next year, your hospital will sponsor a major regional continuing education conference. Your commander gave you an assignment last month to develop a new brochure to promote the conference.

In addition to writing the copy for the brochure, you also were involved in the artwork and production aspects of this project. The photograph that you selected for the cover of the brochure is one that a colleague once gave you, showing a health care team treating a patient. It's very attention-getting and sets the tone for the conference better than anything else you've seen. It reminds you of a Rockwell painting.

This morning, your staff informed you that the first six boxes containing 30 000 brochures had arrived. The brochures cost a total of $18 000, which included art work, layout, paper, and printing. The brochures are extremely convincing and, although you realize this is slightly more than you planned to spend, you believe that this investment will be worth it in terms of attracting a substantial audience.

The brochures look great – better than you ever expected. However, there's a problem: you just noticed that the picture on the front of each brochure is copyrighted by Muffin Studios, a small photography studio in the area. Somehow, you never noticed the copyright before! In a conversation with a coworker, you also just found out that Muffin is assessing a reprint fee of $1 per reproduction of this particular photo. This would cost a total of $30 000 over and above the $18 000 you already paid.

As soon as you realized your mistake, you reported the problem to your commander. The commander advised you to meet today with the President of Muffin Studios with the hope of negotiating an agreement. However, your commander did not tell you what terms to work out. The commander was very angry and simply yelled, "HANDLE IT!"

You called the President of Muffin Studios to set up a meeting. You may not have been too clear on the phone about the purpose of your visit. You simply said, "It's about a photograph you have of a health care team delivering care to a patient, and I would like to talk to you about it in person."

ROLE PLAY: PICTURE PERFECT
CONFIDENTIAL INSTRUCTIONS

President of Muffin Studios

You are the President of Muffin Studios, a small photography studio that has been in business for 10 years. Although Muffin Studios improved its profits during the past two years, there does not seem to be as much business this year. This is of major concern to you because the rent for your studio has just increased and you are still paying off the loan for the state-of-the-art photography equipment you bought last year.

Most of the photography that your company does is for local businesses and industries. One is a picture of health care team delivering care to a patient. Since the photo was taken at a health care facility that no longer exists, you have total ownership of the photograph.

The photograph is a particularly good one; in fact, it is reminiscent of an old Rockwell painting, and it's so good in terms of lighting, composition, etc., that several organizations have expressed an interest in reprinting it. To protect the picture as well as to make a little extra money, you have had this particular photograph copyrighted and decided to assess a $1 fee for every reproduction of the photo.

This morning, you had a call from an official at a well-known VA hospital. The caller simply said, "It's about a photograph you have of a health care team, and I would like to talk to you about it in person." You assume that the caller would like to reproduce the picture, but you are not quite sure. You agreed to a meeting today to discuss it.

Lab work

TYPE: Role play – medical director of a managed care organization and physician leader of a multi-specialty group practice[4]

ESTIMATED TRAINING TIME: 45 minutes

THEME: Negotiation

OBJECTIVE:

➥ to develop skills in negotiations involving relationship and quality issues.

MATERIALS NEEDED: A copy of the General Instructions for all participants, and a copy of the two roles for each dyad

PROCEDURE:

Ask participants to select a partner and distribute the General Instructions to all participants. Then distribute the two roles to each dyad; they will know which role they will play by the sheet they are handed. Point out that there will be a 25-minute time limit for negotiating this exercise, followed by an all-group discussion.

DEBRIEFING:

1 Did the medical director and group practice leader come to an agreement during this discussion? If so, what did they decide to do? Was the practice allowed to carve out lab services from its contract with PrudentCare? Did PrudentCare promise to address the quality issue with the lab? Or did the group practice decide to opt out of its relationship with PrudentCare?

2 If PrudentCare promised to address the quality issue with the lab, will they address all reported problems – not just delayed reports?

3 What was the value of the group practice providing documentation about various problems at Kwik Labs? How would the discussion have differed without such documentation?

4 What was the effect of mentioning the practice's geographic coverage and its relationship with the most prestigious tertiary care teaching hospital in the state?

5 Did it matter that the practice was unhappy about being unable to continue markups on its billing for lab work? Why or why not?

---

4 A special thanks to Gil Weber, MBA, a practice management and managed care consultant for physicians and industry, based in Viera, Florida, for developing the concept of this exercise.

ROLE PLAY: LAB WORK

GENERAL INSTRUCTIONS

PrudentCare, a managed care plan, has decided that its laboratory expenses have been much too high. In the past, physicians who contracted with the plan were allowed to either do lab work in their own offices or send tests to the reference laboratories of their choice. Physicians also were allowed to mark up the lab costs at an attractive margin and bill PrudentCare for the entire amount. Obviously, physicians were receiving most of the benefit from this payment arrangement.

The Chief Financial Officer of PrudentCare decided that this was far too expensive. To reduce costs, the plan has now announced that the plan will begin using a single laboratory, Kwik Labs Inc. In addition, physicians will no longer be able to mark up their lab bills as they did before. Instead, they will have to accept a greatly reduced fee schedule for lab services.

In order to implement the new policy, the Medical Director of PrudentCare is meeting today with the physician leader of a 10-physician multi-specialty practice comprised of family physicians, internists, and pediatricians. The practice has no laboratory in-house. During a phone call earlier this week, the Medical Director of PrudentCare simply told the practice leader about the basics of the new policy, and he/she asked for this meeting to discuss the issue further.

ROLE PLAY: LAB WORK
CONFIDENTIAL INSTRUCTIONS

Medical Director of PrudentCare (Managed Care Plan)

Although you are certain that most physicians in your plan have heard through the grapevine about PrudentCare's intention to have all lab work go through Kwik Labs Inc., this will be your first discussion with any of the physicians in the 10-physician multi-specialty group practice. When you meet with the physician leader of that practice today, you expect some complaining about the doctors having to accept your new fee schedule for lab services, but you believe this matter is up to PrudentCare to decide.

You fully expect that the multi-specialty group practice will stay with PrudentCare. After all, PrudentCare has given a fair amount of business to this practice over the past 10 years, and it is now a very busy and lucrative practice. You are fairly certain that the group will understand that this move is necessary in order for PrudentCare to remain competitive. Kwik Labs Inc. has given your plan rates that are exceptionally reasonable. No other lab could come close.

Your relationship with this multi-specialty group practice is very important to PrudentCare. They are affiliated with the State's most prestigious tertiary care teaching hospital, and the hospital feels very strongly about keeping the group in the network. Another reason this group practice is important is because they have a major presence in a geographic area that is extremely important to your plan.

In the past, the multi-specialty group practice sent their lab tests to two different laboratories (not Kwik Labs Inc.). You believe that Kwik Labs Inc. has acceptable standards and a reasonably good turnaround time. You have heard about some problems that were reported by various users of Kwik Labs Inc., but PrudentCare has been given assurances that corrective measures are being taken to avoid delayed reports.

Your meeting with the physician who leads the group begins now.

ROLE PLAY: LAB WORK
CONFIDENTIAL INSTRUCTIONS

Primary Care Physician

You are the primary care physician managing a 10-physician group. Your practice has been affiliated with PrudentCare for more than 10 years. You have been extremely pleased with most of your dealings with the plan, and believe that your relationship with the plan has been a rewarding one, both personally and professionally. In fact, the business that PrudentCare generates for your group has played a significant role in the growth of your group practice over the years.

Your practice has typically sent laboratory tests to two reference labs, and you have been quite happy with their work. However, you are concerned about doing lab work through Kwik Labs Inc. Ever since your group heard through the grapevine that PrudentCare would require all lab work to be sent to one centralized lab – Kwik Labs Inc. – several of your partners complained and started to collect data about problems with the lab. Working with other practices that have used Kwik Labs Inc. in the past, they were able to document numerous instances of delayed reports, false positives, false negatives, lost specimens, and several other problems that your group finds unacceptable. You plan to present this documentation to the Medical Director of PrudentCare at today's meeting.

From a financial standpoint, you are very concerned about the potential loss of income by being required to use Kwik Labs Inc. and no longer being able to mark up billings for lab work – an especially tough issue now that the group has been hit hard by cuts in Medicare and Medicaid payments – but your concerns about the quality of Kwik Labs Inc. are more distressing to you and your colleagues than anything else.

While you are trying to work out this issue of the quality problems of Kwik Labs Inc. at today's meeting with the Medical Director of PrudentCare, you will stress your practice's strong relationship with the most prestigious hospital in the State and the fact that your practice has a major presence in a geographic area that the plan has worked hard to cover.

Issues involved in
the development
of a medical home
program for your
State

Training Tool #50

The medical home

TYPE: Role play – representatives from Medicaid, State legislature, family medicine association, and nursing association[5]

ESTIMATED TRAINING TIME: 60 minutes

THEMES: Negotiation, conflict management

OBJECTIVES:
➡ to identify issues involved in the establishment of a medical home.
➡ to identify strategies for a multi-party negotiation regarding a new model of care.

MATERIALS NEEDED: A copy of the role play exercise on the next page for all participants

PROCEDURE:
Assemble participants into groups of four and distribute the instruction sheet to everyone. Assign a different role to each person in each group. If there are an uneven number of people, ask extras to double up on a role with another participant or serve as observer. Note that the groups will have 35–40 minutes to negotiate an agreement before reporting on their findings to the group as a whole.

DEBRIEFING:
1 Did this meeting seem more like a negotiation, or a debate? Please explain your response.
2 What were the negotiating points for the family medicine association? For the nursing association?
3 Did the positions of Medicaid and the state legislature work against the family medicine association? Why or why not?
4 How did the previous passage of the Expanded Scope of Practice Act for nurses have a bearing on this discussion?
5 What strategies would make an agreement possible in this situation?

---

5   A special thanks to Rosemarie Sweeney, Vice President of Public Policy and Practice Support of the American Academy of Family Physicians, for developing the concept for this exercise.

ROLE PLAY: THE MEDICAL HOME

You have been meeting for months with various groups to establish a "patient-centered medical home" (PCMH) program in your State. A working definition of the PCMH has been proposed as follows:

> A PCMH is not a building, house, or hospital, but rather an approach to providing comprehensive primary care services in a high-quality and cost-effective manner. Persons who have a PCMH receive the care that they need from a health care team of professionals, **led by a trusted physician.** Health care professionals and patients act as partners in a PCMH to identify and access all medical and non-medical services needed to provide primary care for people of all ages and medical conditions. [Emphasis added.]

When this definition was suggested by the family medicine association, the nurses objected strongly, particularly to language that the PCMH must be physician-led. Today's meeting will be devoted to resolving this issue. Following are the positions of the parties involved in today's meeting:

- **State legislature** – Because the State legislature has passed an Expanded Scope of Practice Act for nurses, independent nursing practices are now legal in this State. As such, the legislature does not see how it can forbid independent nurses from leading a PCMH if nurses are included in the definition.

- **Family medicine association** – This association strongly supports the proposed definition, and is adamant that the PCMH must be physician-led. The association further believes that physicians are best suited to lead PCMHs because of their advanced training and education. They believe that quality of care and the ability of the primary care physician to treat the vast majority of patients' problems, complaints, and conditions are paramount.

- **Nursing association** – This association is vehemently opposed to the proposed definition that requires PCMHs to be physician-led only. The association believes that nurses in independent practices can treat most problems, complaints, and conditions that primary care physicians treat and that referrals by nurses would be at around the same level as primary care physicians' referrals. You resent implications that nurses would not provide the same quality of care.

- **Medicaid** – Your agency must abide by State law, and your State allows independent nursing practice. As such, you believe that whichever professional is the patient's key provider – doctor or nurse – should be able to lead a PCMH. You will support the nurses' definition, but will go along with the group's decision.

Request to hire a
family physician who
does high-risk OB

Training Tool #51

Negotiation at Frugality Hospital

TYPE: Role play – two physicians: Director of Medical Education and Director of the Family Medicine Residency Program

ESTIMATED TRAINING TIME: 60 minutes

THEMES: Negotiation, conflict management

OBJECTIVE:

➡ to identify ways to meet needs in a negotiation involving limited resources.

MATERIALS NEEDED: Copies of the two roles for each dyad

PROCEDURE:

Ask participants to select a partner and distribute a copy of the two roles to each dyad. Announce that the group will have 35 minutes to complete their negotiations and that an all-group discussion will follow.

DEBRIEFING:

1 What were the issues in this scenario?
2 How many that played the role of Dr. Noway agreed to hire Dr. Duitall? Explain your rationale.
3 What other decisions were reached in this discussion?
4 What were Dr. Kinder's responses to Dr. Noway's concerns about expenditures? How did Dr. Kinder handle comments that the residency wasn't bringing in enough revenue?
5 What, if any, were the common needs and interests between these two parties?
6 Did those who played the role of Dr. Noway utilize the extra funds that were available? If so, which considerations led to this decision?

ROLE PLAY: NEGOTIATION AT FRUGALITY HOSPITAL
CONFIDENTIAL INSTRUCTIONS

Dr. Noway, Director of Medical Education

You are an endocrinologist, and have served as the Director of Medical Education at Frugality Hospital for the past three years. Among your many duties, the hospital's four residencies (family medicine, internal medicine, ob-gyn, and surgery) all report to you. You are extremely influential within the hospital; in fact, you often are asked to attend meetings of the hospital Board of Trustees and have noticed that most of the time the Board votes in accordance with your recommendations. You have an excellent rapport with the hospital administrator, particularly since several of your ideas have saved the hospital hundreds of thousands of dollars.

Today you have a meeting with Dr. Kinder, the new Director of the Family Medicine Residency Program. You like Dr. Kinder (who doesn't?) but you don't want to show it too much for fear that he/she will start taking advantage of you. After all, even though Dr. Kinder has been the residency director for only three months, he/she has often talked about changes that should be made to the program to "upgrade it." Although you haven't talked about too many specifics yet, you just know that whatever these changes are will be costly to the hospital. Any change that would cost money at this time – especially in view of the changing political climate and the anticipated loss of some federal funding – is very disturbing to you. After all, you have achieved your clout by being fiscally responsible, and you worry about losing your influence if you don't keep up that image.

You're glad that Dr. Kinder is coming in today, because you need to point out that there will not be any positions available during the next year because the hospital is about to be downsized. Recently, the hospital laid off about 100 employees, and a freeze was placed on full-time equivalents three months ago.

You also want to remind Dr. Kinder that the family medicine residency is not producing nearly enough revenue. Even though the family medicine residency has been doing better since Dr. Kinder came on board, you think this is a fluke and probably won't continue. Besides, you don't think that family medicine will ever bring in as much as the surgical program.

If Dr. Kinder dares to have one of those typical "gimme" attitudes, you'll explain (in your usual brusque style) that there's no room for any new expenditures in the family medicine budget. *[Note: However, if you happen to be swayed by some great rationale or negotiating skills, you do have access to a special fund with $150 000 that the administrator has set aside for emergencies or special purposes.]*

ROLE PLAY: NEGOTIATION AT FRUGALITY HOSPITAL
CONFIDENTIAL INSTRUCTIONS

DR. KINDER, FAMILY MEDICINE RESIDENCY PROGRAM DIRECTOR

You are a new family medicine residency program director; in fact, you were just hired for this position three months ago. Since its inception, the residency program has had very little emphasis on obstetrics, a situation that you plan to change. An impetus to make such changes is a recent Residency Review Committee (RRC) report on your program, which noted that "the number of obstetrical deliveries is low, and there are no family medicine faculty members doing obstetrics."

Last week, you interviewed a candidate for a faculty position (Dr. Duitall) who seems to be an excellent match for your program. Dr. Duitall is a board-certified family physician who has 10 years experience doing a full range of family medicine in a rural community, including high risk OB, and also has faculty experience at a large residency program a few states away. Dr. Duitall is very interested in being affiliated with your residency, and has asked for a minimum of $185 000 per year. You consider this amount quite reasonable in view of Dr. Duitall's qualifications. You are also impressed that Dr. Duitall is willing to perform a minimum of 75 deliveries a year in addition to teaching and supervisory responsibilities.

Today, you will need to seek approval for the new position from your boss, Dr. Noway, an endocrinologist who is the Director of Medical Education at Frugality Hospital. You have not had very pleasant encounters with Dr. Noway thus far, and find him/her to be quite difficult. In the past, you've talked to Dr. Noway in general terms about "upgrading" your residency, but he/she seemed indifferent.

You're hoping that today's discussion will be different. You will try to explain that the obstetricians in town have been overwhelmed by an influx of Medicaid patients, and that your program can help to alleviate this burden. In addition, you will try to get Dr. Noway to understand the importance of addressing problems cited by the RRC, and the financial and other benefits of bringing Dr. Duitall to your program.

The hidden agenda

TYPE: Role play – two physicians and a Board president

ESTIMATED TRAINING TIME: 30 minutes

THEMES: Negotiation, conflict management

OBJECTIVES:
➡ to understand the importance of discerning between people's stated positions and their hidden agendas;
➡ to identify ways to uncover hidden agendas in negotiations, particularly by questioning.

MATERIALS NEEDED: Two copies of the physicians' role and one copy of the Board president's role for each triad

PROCEDURE:
Divide participants into groups of three and distribute the roles so that two are playing the roles of Drs. Ross and Weaver, and the other is the Board president. Allow 15 minutes for the completion of this exercise, and then reconvene for an all-group discussion.

DEBRIEFING:
1 How many layers of hidden agendas did the Board president in your triad get to?
2 Were questions framed in a way that produced the greatest amount of information? How could the questions have been framed differently?
3 Was getting to the hidden agenda easier or more difficult by dealing with both Drs. Ross and Weaver at once?
4 Why would it be easier for the physicians to ask for the pay increase, the bonuses, and inclusion at Board meetings rather than say what they *really* wanted?
5 How did Ms. Lockhart say she'd address the doctors' real needs? What would have to happen so that Drs. Ross and Weaver would know that their needs were being met?

ROLE PLAY: THE HIDDEN AGENDA
GENERAL INSTRUCTIONS

Drs. Ross and Weaver have been providing primary care services at County Community Health Center for the past five years. When the doctors were asked to commit to another three years at the center, they said they had some demands that would need to be addressed first, e.g. more compensation.

When the administrator, Ms. Romano, asked if the physicians would agree to stay if she agreed to their demands for higher salaries and bonuses, the doctors acted reluctant to commit. Ms. Romano said they were being bullheaded and asked, "Are you maneuvering to try to get me to go even higher on the amounts? Is that why you're acting this way?"

The doctors said that they were too angry to continue the discussion, and said they'd like to speak to the president of the center's Community Board of Directors, Ms. Lockhart.

"Well, I can't stop you," Ms. Romano said. "But you should be dealing directly with me on this matter."

Several days have passed and Ms. Lockhart is about to meet with Drs. Ross and Weaver to try to convince them to stay.

ROLE PLAY: THE HIDDEN AGENDA
CONFIDENTIAL INSTRUCTIONS

Drs. Ross and Weaver

Although the person playing the role of Ms. Lockhart, the Board president, doesn't know it, it will not be possible for either of you to reveal your hidden agendas unless she asks you questions that would cause you to do so if this were a real life situation. At each level, try to show that there is something else on your mind, but be a bit reluctant to reveal more until the right questions are asked. If the questions wouldn't cause you to reveal more, keep repeating information you have already given.

What you will let Ms. Lockhart know right away:

▶ You both want an additional $12000 added to each of your salaries, and a productivity bonus of $10000 per year. You feel that this is very much deserved, as you are now both working during some evenings (you only worked days when your original contracts were signed) and you are also now sharing call at a local long-term care facility.

▶ Getting these increases will increase the likelihood that you will both stay at the health center, but will not assure it.

If good questions are asked, reveal these points:

▶ Neither of you have had good working relationships with the center's administrator, Ms. Romano. She does not consult with you on matters that you believe require physician input. She does not keep you in the loop; you often do not hear about things that are happening until you hear it from a nurse or a member of the front-office staff. She calls you by your first names in front of patients and staff, despite your protests. And she treats you both like she treats the rest of the staff – poorly.

▶ Although the center's administrator is always invited, you have not been included in meetings of the center's Community Board of Directors unless there is an issue that concerns you and your partner directly. You believe that physicians should be present and have input on all matters affecting the center, not just clinically-related matters.

If more good questions are asked, reveal your real hidden agenda:

▶ What you both really want – and what would make you both agree to stay – is more respect from both the administrator and the Board.

ROLE PLAY: THE HIDDEN AGENDA
CONFIDENTIAL INSTRUCTIONS

Ms. Lockhart, Board President

As President of the Community Board of Directors of County Community Health Center, you want to be as helpful as you can to the medical staff as they are at the heart of the center's success. You are very happy with Drs. Weaver and Ross, two outstanding physicians who have been providing primary care services at the center for the past five years. They have been doing a lot of extra work lately, and during the past year, they've even worked some evenings for the sake of employed patients and also have been sharing call at a local long-term care facility.

You recently received a call from the two physicians asking you to meet with them to discuss the continuation of their contract. You asked why they weren't discussing this matter with Ms. Romano, the center's administrator, but they said they would rather talk to you.

While you find it odd that you've been pulled into this discussion, the Board ultimately will have to approve any changes in the doctors' contracts so you might as well hear about their concerns now. You have already heard that they want a salary increase and a productivity bonus. You have already discussed this with the Board, and they will have no problem with this as long as the request is reasonable.

Above all, you want the doctors to stay in the community, so it's important to you to address their concerns and ensure that they are as happy with the Center as the Board and entire community are with them.

Your meeting with Drs. Ross and Weaver begins now.

Dealing with difficult colleagues

Reflecting on a difficult behavior

TYPE: Introductory discussion

ESTIMATED TRAINING TIME: 30 minutes

THEMES: Difficult colleagues, conflict management, negotiation

OBJECTIVE:

➡ to dissect the manner in which participants have handled colleagues with difficult behaviors in the past in order to learn from those experiences.

MATERIALS NEEDED: A copy of the discussion sheet on the following page for all participants

PROCEDURE:

Break into groups of three and distribute a copy of the discussion sheet to everyone. Point out that the members of each group will be asked to describe a difficult behavior that they have personally encountered with a colleague in a health care setting and to answer the questions on the discussion sheet. Point out that no names should be used; even if the individual is not likely to be known by others, it's a small enough world that someone still might know them.

Each individual in the small groups should take 10 minutes each to answer the questions on the sheet and receive input and suggestions from other group members.

Describe a situation you have experienced involving a difficult colleague.

1 Who was involved? (Describe individuals by roles, professions, and demographics, not by name – even if the situation occurred long ago in a different health care organization.)

2 What did that individual do that presented a problem? Was this a chronic problem or isolated event?

3 What are possible reasons for this person's behavior? (Don't just demonize the other party; give them the benefit of the doubt.)

4 At which party was the behavior directed?

5 When and how did you realize that this behavior was adversely affecting you, your colleagues, and/or your health care organization?

6 What was *your* role in perpetuating this person's behavior?

7 What were this individual's good qualities?

8 How did you initially react to the problem behavior?

9 What strategies did you apply?

10 Were your interventions effective? If not, what other steps did you take?

11 What would you do differently when encountering similar behaviors in the future?

12 What is the "take away" lesson from this discussion?

Dealing with difficult behaviors

TYPE: Worksheet

ESTIMATED TRAINING TIME: 30 minutes

THEMES: Difficult colleagues, conflict management, negotiation

OBJECTIVES:

➡ to identify participants' tendencies, feelings, and opinions about dealing with difficult behaviors;

➡ to show that it's not always the other person who is difficult – sometimes, it's us!

MATERIALS NEEDED: A copy of the worksheet on the following page for all participants

PROCEDURE:

Tell participants they will have 15 minutes to fill out the worksheet. Point out that for this exercise to have value, it's important to be as honest and introspective as possible.

DEBRIEFING:

After 15 minutes, tell the group that they will not have to disclose their responses unless they are willing to, but that sharing this information will help to increase understanding about one another's tendencies and opinions about dealing with difficult behaviors. (To make it easier for others to share the information from their worksheets, the instructor may wish to start by sharing his/her own.)

Worksheet

1 When I'm dealing with difficult behaviors and situations, my greatest fear is that I'll . . .

2 The type of difficult behavior that bothers me the most is when people . . .

3 I usually deal with that behavior by . . .

4 Some of my "hot buttons" (words or actions that "set me off") include:

5 When someone presses my hot buttons, I normally . . .

6 My own difficult behaviors include . . .

7 When others point out my difficult behaviors, I normally react by . . .

8 When my behavior has been difficult, it has usually occurred when (because) . . .

9 If I could wave a magic wand and get some of my colleagues to behave differently, they would . . .

10 I've been most successful in dealing with difficult behaviors when I . . .

Sticks and stones

TYPE: Case study

ESTIMATED TRAINING TIME: 30 minutes

THEMES: Difficult colleagues, emotional intelligence

OBJECTIVE:

➡ to develop strategies for dealing with a health care professional's anger problem.

MATERIALS NEEDED: A copy of the case study on the following page for all participants

PROCEDURE:

Distribute the case study to all participants and give them a few minutes to read and analyze it.

DEBRIEFING:

1 Who is the person with the difficult behavior – the physician, the nurse, or both? Explain your response.
2 Was the nurse justified in being offended, whether or not she made these errors?
3 If the nurse did make the errors, would that excuse the doctor for the way he handled these situations? Why or why not?
4 Taking this situation at face value, what are some possible reasons for the doctor's anger? Were the actions taken to deal with the doctor enough? What actions, if any, should be taken in regard to the nurse's performance?
5 Does the physician sound like a good doctor who cares about his patients? Why or why not?
6 If you are coaching this doctor, what would you suggest to him?
7 What, if anything, could be done to repair the working relationship between the doctor and the nurse? What can be done by the two individuals? By the anesthesiology department? By the nursing division? By administration?
8 What are the lessons from this case about interpersonal communication and professionalism?

CASE STUDY: STICKS AND STONES

I've been an anesthesiologist at this oceanside medical center on the west coast for more than 30 years now, and I'll never apologize to anyone about my standards of excellence. I've had these values all of my professional life, and that I'm almost 60, I'm quite set in my ways. I get along with most people, and I don't have any communication or relationship problems with the nurses that I like, but I simply have no tolerance for incompetence.

There's one nurse at work who is the most incompetent person I've ever known. I'll give you a couple of examples. A few weeks ago, this nurse allowed air to get into a critical patient's blood line in the emergency room. I screamed at her, "YOU INCOMPETENT *##* YOU'RE KILLING THE PATIENT!" I pointed to the door and told her to get out NOW. She left. I handled things from there, and thank God, the patient made it.

Another time, she was with me in the ER and I was trying to revive a patient so I told her to move. She wouldn't get out of the way fast enough, so I called her an idiot. She just stood there when I called her that, so I had no choice; I literally had to push her aside.

Okay, now here's the part you're not going to believe. Here's this stupid idiot nurse who jeopardizes patients' lives, and yet she reports *me* to administration and I'm the one who gets written up! I was telling the other docs in my department how incompetent she is and that we've got to get rid of her, but they say it's not up to us and that they haven't had anything bad happen when they've worked with her. Some even said she was one of our best nurses, and I don't get that at all.

Administration wants me to formally apologize for embarrassing her and calling her names. They said what I did was unprofessional. It's unreal . . . she's incompetent, I'm the one saving lives, yet I'm the one who gets written up! Go figure.

The e-tantrum

TYPE: Case study

ESTIMATED TRAINING TIME: 15 minutes

THEME: Difficult colleagues

OBJECTIVES:

➡ to understand that people can inadvertently come across as "difficult" by the way they write emails;

➡ to develop skills in writing and utilizing emails effectively and efficiently.

MATERIALS NEEDED: A copy of the case study on the following pages for all participants

PROCEDURE:

Distribute the case study on the following pages and give participants a minute or two to identify the good and bad points about the messages and how they are written.

DEBRIEFING:

1 What, if anything, is good about this exchange of emails?

2 Was it understandable that Ms. Thyme interpreted the email as "being yelled at in writing"? If so, what was it about Dr. Shepherd's emails that led to this perception?

3 What were the other problems with this exchange of emails?

4 Did it seem that Ms. Thyme was addressing the doctor's orders, or was she more concerned about whether she was in trouble?

5 What could Dr. Shepherd have done differently to deal with this issue?

6 Should emails be used in a situation like this? When is face-to-face communication more appropriate?

7 What are the lessons from this case about emails in the workplace?

CASE STUDY: THE E-TANTRUM

From: Darrin Shepherd, MD
To: Justina Thyme
Subject: Problem

Ms. Thyme

I just learned that you have scheduled me for a 4:00 pm appointment today. I expressly said that I DID NOT want any appointments today scheduled past 3:30 pm. **WHAT ABOUT THIS DIRECTIVE DID YOU NOT UNDERSTAND?**

Dr. Shepherd

From: Justina Thyme
To: Darrin Shepherd, MD
Subject: Problem

Hi Dr. Shepherd

I'm so sorry! But what happened is that I got a call from your patient, Brittany Shears, and she sounded so terrible that I felt it was necessary to work her into your schedule. I knew you didn't have to be at your meeting tonight until 5:00 pm, so I figured this would be all right.

Justina ☺

From: Darrin Shepherd, MD
To: Justina Thyme
Subject: Problem

Ms. Thyme

Ms. Shears has an appointment with me next week, so if the problem couldn't have waited until then, she needs to go to the ER.

    I do not believe you understand the problem. When you work patients into the schedule, **YOU MUST CONSULT ME FIRST!**

Dr. Shepherd

Hi Dr. Shepherd

Normally I would have done that, but we looked for you and couldn't find you when Brittany called. I couldn't say I'd call her back because she was calling from her cell phone and her battery was going out. She really did sound like she was in a lot of pain. Hope you aren't too mad at me!

Justina ☺

MS. THYME

RESCHEDULE MS. SHEAR'S APPOINTMENT AS I HAVE INSTRUCTED.

Darrin Shepherd, MD

From: Justina Thyme
To: Patricia Place
Subject: You won't believe it!

Hey Pat

I'm so upset that I thought I'd write and tell you what's going on!

Remember that awful doctor I was telling you about, Dr. Shepherd? Well, he's been on my back ALL morning! A patient called and she said she was in terrible pain and was crying, so I worked her in for an appointment at 4:00 pm. The doctor had told me not to schedule anyone after 3:30, but I had to make a quick decision because this girl Brittany Shear's cell phone was going out. I KNOW I did the right thing to schedule her in!

What a total jerk Dr. Shepherd is – he's ticked off that I didn't "obey" him so he's been sending me nasty emails, like he's yelling at me in writing! He's the rudest doctor I've ever worked for. I can't believe he doesn't put his patients first.

Well, that's my day . . . how's yours?

XXXXOOOO

Justina ☹

From: Darrin Shepherd, MD
To: Justina Thyme
Subject: MAJOR PROBLEM

Ms. Thyme

I have received your recent email to Ms. Patricia Place, obviously sent to me by mistake. See me immediately.

Dr. Shepherd

Better late than never

TYPE: Case study

ESTIMATED TRAINING TIME: 30 minutes

THEMES: Difficult colleagues, conflict management

OBJECTIVES:

➡ to understand how colleagues can be perceived as difficult when not attending to others' needs;

➡ to describe ways that relationships can be repaired after a difficult situation or encounter.

MATERIALS NEEDED: A copy of the case study on the following page for all participants

PROCEDURE:

Assemble participants into groups of four or five, and assign them the case study that appears on the next page. Note that they will have 15 minutes to assess the nature of the problem and develop recommendations.

DEBRIEFING:

1 Which party or parties were exhibiting the "difficult" behaviors in this case: Dr. Demon, the entire staff, or both?

2 Did it seem that Dr. Demon and the staff saw themselves as difficult? Why or why not?

3 Did the behaviors seem to be purposeful or inadvertent?

4 What could have been done or said to have avoided Dr. Affect's feeling that he was disenfranchised from his own practice?

5 What issues were involved in this case?

6 What could be done to repair the relationship between Drs. Affect and Demon?

CASE STUDY: BETTER LATE THAN NEVER

Drs. Ben Affect and Matt Demon met during their first year of medical school and soon became best friends. Their families went on several vacations together and often socialized on evenings and holidays. After attending the same family medicine residency program, Drs. Affect and Demon decided to go into practice together. When they learned that a well-equipped health center in a small rural town was looking for two family physicians with similar practice styles to replace a beloved physician who had retired after 35 years of practice, they jumped at the chance.

Because Dr. Affect had already signed up for a post-residency fellowship in geriatrics, they agreed that Dr. Demon would begin to practice by himself and Dr. Affect would join him six months later.

Nurses and other staff members at the health center built a strong bond with Dr. Demon immediately. To mark his arrival, they displayed a huge welcome banner in the office and presented him with cards and notes. The administrator threw a party in his honor, with a "Who's Who" of community leaders in attendance. As the only physician in the health center for the next six months, Dr. Demon felt a little stressed from the high patient load and often wished that Dr. Affect had been there to help out. Even so, Dr. Demon and the staff were blissfully content.

As soon as Dr. Affect completed his fellowship, he eagerly came to the health center to begin practice with Dr. Demon. Unlike his partner, Dr. Affect received a lukewarm reception. There was no banner and no party. Except for assigning a large number of patients to Dr. Affect, Dr. Demon went on with his practice as if nothing was different. He acted a little annoyed when Dr. Affect did anything differently, and frequently gave him a series of "lectures" about how he had reorganized the practice and how it now functioned. As he had done for the past six months, Dr. Demon led each staff meeting. Dr. Affect began to worry about his relationships with staff. He often saw Dr. Demon in hallways sharing in-jokes with staff members. When Dr. Affect asked clinicians and staff members to follow certain procedures, most sought approval from Dr. Demon first.

Feeling that he had very little voice or support, Dr. Affect decided to meet with Dr. Demon. He explained that while Dr. Demon had created a solid team, the team was not letting him in! "It's just a matter of timing," Dr. Demon responded. "Things will be okay when the staff gets to know you." Dr. Demon left, saying he had something else to do.

Dr. Affect sank into his chair. He thought, "What can I do to fit into this team when my own partner doesn't care?"

The Mount Vesuvius effect

TYPE: Case study

ESTIMATED TRAINING TIME: 30 minutes

THEMES: Difficult colleagues, conflict management, negotiation, emotional intelligence

OBJECTIVE:

➡ to identify ways to deal with a colleague's passive-aggressive behavior.

MATERIALS NEEDED: A copy of the case study on the following page for all participants

PROCEDURE:

Explain that the Mount Vesuvius effect[6] is what happens when an individual keeps emotions bottled up inside and tensions pile up, one on top of the other; ultimately, the emotions "explode" when the person reaches his/her personal threshold.

Give the group a few minutes to read the case study and ask the following questions.

DEBRIEFING:

1 What are some of the likely reasons that Dr. Lusion lost her temper? Did the weeks of holding back her feelings have any bearing on this?

2 Does it seem that Dr. Lusion was aware of the intensity of her feelings in her early conversations about the advanced medical home program with her partners? Please explain.

3 What are the effects of Dr. Lusion's outbursts on her colleagues? On the office atmosphere?

4 What can Drs. Cheever and Patienz do about this situation? What strategies are most likely to work if this occurred in real life?

---

6 Author's note: I read about the "Mount Vesuvius effect" in a textbook many years ago, and while the concept has stayed with me, I cannot find the source. Whoever coined this phrase, thank you – and let me know who you are! EJB

CASE STUDY: THE MOUNT VESUVIUS EFFECT

Eva Lusion, MD, has been in private group practice with two partners, Dr. Seymour Patienz and Iman H. Cheever, for the past two years. Dr. Lusion is normally quite low-key, but occasionally has disagreements with her two partners about the way the practice should be run. She is described by her partners as being very personable, yet often quite shy and reserved.

One of Dr. Lusion's partners, Dr. Cheever, regularly attends medical meetings where she gets a lot of ideas that she wants to implement. For example, just lately she proposed that the group become part of the State's new advanced medical home program. This would require the practice to install an electronic medical record (EMR) system, and develop a way to track laboratory results and referrals. It will mean a whole new culture for the practice – and numerous additional expenses.

When Dr. Cheever asked her partners to join the advanced medical home program, Dr. Patienz agreed immediately.

"This is going to make a huge difference in our ability to provide the type of primary care services that we've always wanted," Dr. Patienz said, "and we'll be able to treat entire populations!"

Dr. Lusion sat quietly while her two partners excitedly discussed the possibilities for their practice by affiliating with the advanced medical home program. However, inside she was deeply concerned about how much time it would take for her to learn the EMR system. It also bothered her to think that she would be responsible for developing the tracking systems because she had more skills in this area than her partners. She decided not to comment about her concerns, because she didn't want to put a damper on her partners' enthusiasm. Besides, she wanted to think about it more.

For the next week or so, every time Drs. Patienz and Cheever saw Dr. Lusion in the hallways or at the front desk, they would urge her to "join the bandwagon."

"We can't do this unless *all* of us agree to it, Eva. You're the only one holding us up." At times, they would joke with her about her indecision; at other times, they would act frustrated and disappointed. Their pressure on Dr. Lusion was relentless.

When Dr. Cheever called for another partners' meeting to discuss the issue, the meeting had barely begun when Dr. Lusion began to shout.

"I HAVE HAD IT WITH YOU BOTH! I CAN'T TAKE THE TIME TO LEARN EMR! I KNOW YOU'LL HAVE ME DO THE LAB AND REFERRAL TRACKING, SO I'LL BE DOING MORE THAN BOTH YOU OF COMBINED . . . AS USUAL!"

"Whoa," Dr. Patienz said. "Where in the world did this come from? All you had to do was tell us about your concerns, Eva. We'd share the responsibilities . . ."

Flushed with anger – and perhaps embarrassment from her meltdown – Dr. Lusion stormed out of the conference room and slammed the door.

"We're going to have to walk on eggshells again," said Dr. Cheever. "Each time this happens, she doesn't tell us what she's been thinking and then, out of nowhere, she explodes."

"I know what you mean," Dr. Patienz said. "And each explosion seems to get worse than the last."

A physician and
nurse argue about
his involvement in a
prenatal project

Training Tool #59

Oyl and Water

TYPE: Case study

ESTIMATED TRAINING TIME: 30 minutes

THEMES: Difficult colleagues, conflict management

OBJECTIVES:

➡ to show how a grudge match can turn valuable employees into persons with "difficult behaviors;"

➡ to identify ways to resolve issues among two difficult parties.

MATERIALS NEEDED: A copy of the case study on the following page for all participants

PROCEDURE:

Assemble participants into groups of four to five people, and give them a few minutes to review the case study. Note that they will have 15 minutes to assess the nature of the problem and develop recommendations.

DEBRIEFING:

1 What difficult behaviors are evident in this case?
2 Is one party more responsible for this problem than the other? Why or why not? Does it even matter who is responsible?
3 What are Dr. Oyl and Ms. Water doing that is not working? What are they doing that might be perpetuating this problem?
4 What strategies can be applied to deal with this situation?
5 What is the effect of their poor working relationship on other staff members?
6 How did you feel about the MCH director's action to turn this problem back to the individuals involved?
7 If the discussion between Dr. Oyl and Ms. Water doesn't result in improvements, what other steps might be taken?

CASE STUDY: OYL AND WATER

Vincent Oyl, MD, a pediatrician, and Beth Water, RN, a public health nurse, both work in the Maternal and Child Health (MCH) Division of a State Department of Health. Dr. Oyl and Ms. Water have worked together on several projects and have similar job titles. Their working relationship started to break down a few months ago.

The problem started when Dr. Oyl insisted on getting involved in a project to coordinate a series of immunization clinics for children in a medium-sized community. Although Ms. Water had been in charge of this project for nearly two years, Dr. Oyl started to make numerous suggestions on how the project should be changed so that she can extend the boundaries of the project to include another county.

From Ms. Water's perspective, this is none of Dr. Oyl's business. After all, he is not even assigned to the immunization project! Ms. Water believes that the doctor's suggestions would make her work much more complicated. She wonders, "Does he realize that we are extremely short staffed and working more than 60 hours a week?" Although Ms. Water became quite angry, she didn't tell Dr. Oyl directly. Instead, she started to act rudely toward the doctor and made several negative comments about Dr. Oyl to her nursing colleagues.

Dr. Oyl knows that Ms. Water is upset, but he's not quite sure why. He knows that Ms. Water has said terrible things about him behind his back, for example, calling him a "control freak." Except for referring to Ms. Water as a "moody little girl," Dr. Oyl believes that he is relatively blameless for this situation, especially in regard to the immunization project. He thought his suggestions would be helpful!

Because Ms. Water is treating him so terribly these days, Dr. Oyl either avoids her or makes snide comments. Now the relationship between Dr. Oyl and Ms. Water is so strained that others are uncomfortable in their presence. When the MCH director found out about this, she called Dr. Oyl and Ms. Water into her office. "This is not acceptable," the director said. "This is not setting a good example for other staff members, and you've both demoralized and upset others. I insist that you meet to work out your differences."

An associate hospital
administrator rips up
a meeting agenda

Training Tool #60

Jack the Ripper

TYPE: Case study

ESTIMATED TRAINING TIME: 30 minutes

THEMES: Difficult colleagues, conflict management, emotional intelligence

OBJECTIVE:

➡ to determine ways to deal with a colleague's disruptive outburst.

MATERIALS NEEDED: A copy of the case study on the following page for all participants

PROCEDURE:
After discussing ways to deal with outbursts and other difficult behaviors, give the group a few minutes to review the case study and ask the debriefing questions.

DEBRIEFING:
1   What was the likely reason for Mr. Ripper's frustration with the process?
2   How should Ms. Peacely address Mr. Ripper's concerns? Should she mention the hard work that went into developing the agenda? Should she discard the agenda and address what is most important to Mr. Ripper? Why or why not?
3   Would it be a good idea for Ms. Peacely (or others) to help Mr. Ripper to save face? If so, what could be done or said to do that?
4   What could be done to neutralize the emotional intensity in the room?
5   Would it be best if Mr. Ripper left the session? If not, what could be done to encourage him to stay?

CASE STUDY: JACK THE RIPPER

The State health department is responsible for administering a grant to develop comprehensive perinatal services in the State. In the northwestern part of the State, the cooperation of three hospitals is essential to the project's implementation. Because of major disagreements between the three hospitals in that area regarding their respective responsibilities in this project, the department has refused to release funding to the hospitals until the dispute is resolved. Unfortunately, the dispute has been going on for three years.

The department called for a meeting to resolve the dispute and put together an extensive agenda so that there could be a free-flowing discussion about the issues that are causing the greatest contention. The Director of Family Health Services, Paula Peacely, worked on this agenda for weeks, and was very proud of how she organized it. Each agenda item was placed strategically in order to ensure that the discussion would move easily from one topic to the next. Several appendices were added to give the group the data they needed to come to a decision.

One of the attendees at this meeting was Jack Ripper, an Associate Administrator at Luzingdough Hospital. When some of his colleagues sat between representatives of the other two hospitals, Mr. Ripper went to each of them and insisted that they all sit together. They did, although some moved reluctantly.

Ms. Peacely distributed the agenda to all participants and expressed the department's hope that the agenda would help lead to a resolution so that the funding could be dispersed and the project could get underway as soon as possible. She smiled broadly, fully expecting that the group would be impressed by her hard work on developing what she referred to as her "beautiful agenda." It was so good and so detailed, she suspected even Henry Kissinger would commend her for it!

Within a moment or two, Mr. Ripper's face turned red as he flipped through the pages. "I AM NOT GOING TO FOLLOW THIS STUPID AGENDA!" he pronounced. He ripped it in two and threw the pieces on the table. "YOU DON'T EVEN ADDRESS THE FUNDING ISSUE UNTIL THE THIRD ITEM ON THE AGENDA – AND THAT'S WHAT WE'RE HERE TO DISCUSS!"

Ms. Peacely's mouth dropped open in surprise, and others around the room had varying reactions. Some nodded in agreement; others acted disturbed by Mr. Ripper's behavior. As Mr. Ripper stood up, preparing to leave, the tension in the room was palpable. Ms. Peacely realized that she had to think quickly to determine how to address Mr. Ripper's concerns so that the meeting could continue.

A physician assistant
invents a reference
source to make a
point

Training Tool #61

Questionable source

TYPE: Case study

ESTIMATED TRAINING TIME: 30 minutes

THEMES: Difficult colleagues, difficult conversations

OBJECTIVE:

➡ to identify ways of dealing with a colleague who occasionally stretches the truth.

MATERIALS NEEDED: A copy of the case study on the following page for all participants

PROCEDURE:

In a brief discussion, address the pressures upon health care professionals to be "right" in clinical matters, and how this pressure may extend into other areas as well. Ask the group if they know people who have an aversion to the phrase "I don't know" or those who have great difficulty admitting when they're wrong or mistaken. Then ask, "What problems can result from this? To what lengths will these persons go to win their arguments?"

Give participants a few minutes to read the case, and then ask the following questions.

DEBRIEFING:

1 What are some likely reasons why Ms. Ino became defensive?
2 How would you evaluate how the doctor handled this situation?
3 Would it have been a good idea for the doctor to have helped Ms. Ino save face in this instance? Why or why not?
4 What are appropriate responses when you suspect that a colleague isn't being straight with you or is deliberately giving you erroneous information? How would you handle a situation differently if a colleague gave you erroneous information inadvertently? How would you know if it was deliberate or not?
5 What can be changed in the practice's culture to make it easier for health care professionals to admit mistakes or what they don't know?

CASE STUDY: A QUESTIONABLE SOURCE

Dr. Anita Teechya took Shirley Ino, physician assistant, aside to discuss a recent patient complaint.

"I just heard from one of your patients, Joe Aking, who had a problem with your last visit with him. I thought we should discuss it," Dr. Teechya said.

"I know exactly what this is about," replied Ms. Ino. "Joe is always looking for hand-holding."

"Well, he did just find out that he has liver disease," Dr. Teechya said. "Maybe he's seeking a little compassion."

Ms. Ino sat down and explained, "I don't believe in pampering patients. Some people spend their lives abusing their bodies – just as he did – and then they want me to baby them and say that everything is okay. That's not my style."

Dr. Teechya looked sternly at Ms. Ino. "I'm not saying that you should, Shirley. But I am saying that you could demonstrate empathy for what the patient is going through."

"I know what I'm doing," Ms. Ino said. "In fact, there's an article in the *New England Journal of Medicine* that says that patients have better outcomes when they aren't coddled."

"Well, I've been reading the journal regularly for years," Dr. Teechya noted, looking at Ms. Ino dubiously. "There has never been such an article."

"Are you calling me a liar?" Ms. Ino asked.

"Well, tell me," said Dr. Teechya. "Which issue was the article in? What was the title? Who was the author?"

Ms. Ino stood and headed toward the door. "I'll bring it in when I can find it," she said. "For now, I've got work to do."

A physician who
berates others is
quite valuable to a
group practice

Training Tool #62

The Wright stuff

TYPE: Case study

ESTIMATED TRAINING TIME: 30 minutes

THEMES: Difficult colleagues, conflict management

OBJECTIVE:

➡ to identify ways to convince an effective but difficult colleague to change behaviors.

MATERIALS NEEDED: A copy of the case study on the following page for all participants

PROCEDURE:

Assemble participants into groups of four or five, and assign them to review the case study that appears on the next page. Note that they will have 25 minutes to assess the nature of the problem and develop recommendations before the group reconvenes for an all-group discussion.

DEBRIEFING:

1 What difficult behaviors are apparent in this scenario? Is Dr. Wright the only one responsible for this problem? Why or why not?
2 In terms of "sides" to this issue, how does the 14 to 1 ratio affect the group's ability to deal with Dr. Wright? Which parties should be involved in dealing with this problem – the entire group or selected representatives?
3 What is the group currently doing that's not helping the situation?
4 What strategies would work best in dealing with Dr. Wright – keeping in mind that the group is highly dependent on his extraordinary skills?
5 What communication tips would you recommend?
6 Since people admit that Dr. Wright is extremely effective in getting things done, what is his incentive to change behaviors?
7 How can the group avoid similar problems in the future?

CASE STUDY: THE WRIGHT STUFF

Dr. IM Wright began to practice at Wellville Group Practice 12 years ago. He is one of the senior partners of this multi-specialty group comprised of 15 physicians.

Dr. Wright takes great pride in having superior accounting and business skills and plays a major role in helping the group remain financially viable. Even though he is no longer an officer in the group, Dr. Wright is perceived to have more authority than the president and administrator of the group combined. He has the greatest influence on all of the clinic's financial matters and few decisions are made without consulting Dr. Wright first.

Members of the group are getting increasingly upset about Dr. Wright's behavior. Some are upset when Dr. Wright jokingly says, "My colleagues are clueless about financial matters," even though they secretly agree with him. The five female physicians are upset with several insensitive remarks that Dr. Wright made when they asked to work fewer hours in order to spend more time with their children. Others are simply upset that Dr. Wright's controlling behavior is impeding their ability to function as a team. Some refer to him as a bully.

Dr. Wright is the first to speak up at meetings, always has an opinion, and nearly always opposes change. The clinic's relationship with the local hospital has nearly broken down, and most people attribute this to Dr. Wright's personality. (He recently called the hospital administrator "a liar" to his face.) About three months ago, the president had a few words with Dr. Wright about his behavior. Dr. Wright laughed and said he couldn't change. When he pointed out that he is extremely effective in getting things done, the president couldn't help but agree.

Other than the president, none of the other physicians at the clinic have voiced concerns directly to Dr. Wright – only behind his back. Tensions within the clinic are beginning to grow now that a major expansion is underway.

Difficult conversations

Challenging conversations

TYPE: Introductory discussion

ESTIMATED TRAINING TIME: 15 minutes

THEME: Difficult conversations

OBJECTIVE:

➡ to introduce the subject of challenging or difficult conversations in health care.

MATERIALS NEEDED: Flip chart, optional

PROCEDURE:
Following an overview of the inevitability of difficult conversations in health care situations, ask the group the following questions.

DEBRIEFING:
1 What difficult conversations are most common in health care settings? What are the most difficult types of conversations to have with one's colleagues?
2 What makes these interactions particularly difficult?
3 While these conversations are hard for those on the receiving end, what are the emotional effects on those delivering the information?
4 What communication skills are most essential for handling these difficult conversations?
5 Since these conversations are always difficult by nature, does practice and experience make a difference? If so, how?

Training Tools #64–9

Practicing difficult conversations

TYPE: Case studies

ESTIMATED TRAINING TIME: 30 minutes

THEME: Difficult conversations

OBJECTIVE:

➥ to develop skills in handling various types of difficult conversations involving colleagues, patients, family members, and others.

MATERIALS NEEDED: A copy of two selected cases for all participants

PROCEDURE:

Distribute two selected cases from the following pages and discuss the cases in all-group or small-group discussions. Ask participants to consider what they would do or say to handle each matter as effectively as possible. If additional time is available, select more cases. Your choices are as follows:

➥ **A hairy problem** – Tell a defensive mother to take extra measures to treat her child's head lice.

➥ **Added stress** – Ask a school nurse to handle two additional schools at no extra pay.

➥ **Motor mouth** – Deal with a nurse who tends to over-explain when asked a question.

➥ **Lay off** – Tell a beloved, long-term employee that she will be laid off from her job.

➥ **Adding insult to injury** – Talk to a patient who left her last doctor for calling her "fat."

➥ **Dress code** – Discuss dress codes with a long-haired doctor with a nose ring.

Ask participants to address the questions following each case, as well as any other questions that occur to them.

CASE STUDY: A HAIRY PROBLEM

You need to tell a belligerent mother that her child still has head lice and that she needs to take additional measures to treat this problem at home. All other cases of head lice in the school have been eradicated, and this is the only child who still has the problem.

The mother insists that she has done everything that has been recommended and believes that her child is being re-infected in school. The mother is highly insulted that she is being blamed for this problem, after all of her efforts to take care of it.

DISCUSSION QUESTIONS

1 Is it important to find out the reason that this child continues to have head lice? Why or why not?
2 Why do you think the mother is embarrassed about this problem?
3 How will you assure the mother that the issue isn't about blaming, but to take care of her child's problem?
4 If it turned out that something the mother was or wasn't doing was contributing to the continuation of the child's head lice, how would you address the issue then?
5 How would you deal with the mother's belligerence and defensiveness?

CASE STUDY: ADDED STRESS

You are just about to sit down with a school nurse to point out that, due to budget cuts, she needs to provide services at two more schools. Unfortunately, there will be no increase in pay. This nurse, who already is the school nurse at two other schools, feels that she is overworked already. You are aware that the nurse, a widow with two children, has recently refinanced the mortgage on her home because of one of her children's extensive medical bills.

DISCUSSION QUESTIONS

1   How would you set the tone for this conversation? Would you preface your remarks? If so, how?
2   Would you mention what you know about the nurse's current personal problems? Is that relevant to this situation? Please explain.
3   How can you best deal with the news that there is no additional pay available for the extra responsibilities?
4   Assuming that there is no choice for the nurse other than to accept the new responsibilities or leave her job, what can you do or say that will help the nurse to adapt to this new circumstance?

CASE STUDY: MOTOR MOUTH

It seems that every time you ask one of your nurses a question to find out what's going on, she tends to over-explain. Just the other day, you asked her if a meeting had been scheduled for the medical center's quality improvement conference, and she told you about every conversation and every plan she made to prepare for it, including what she decided to serve for the meal functions. All you wanted was a simple yes or no! This happens nearly every time you talk with her, so you find yourself avoiding her unless there's something you absolutely must know.

You need to ask her today how many persons have signed up for the conference, and your computer has crashed so there's no option other than asking her. You know this will tie you up for a lot longer than you'd like and you're dreading the discussion.

DISCUSSION QUESTIONS

1 How do the two parties differ in terms of the amount of information they prefer to exchange? How do they differ in the use of their time?

2 What are some possible reasons why the nurse tends to over-explain herself? How might she perceive the reasons for your questions about her activities?

3 Will you start out by asking the question about how many people will attend the conference – or will you preface your remarks by instructing her to be brief?

4 How could you let the nurse know that you need briefer responses to simple questions without quelling her enthusiasm? Would you do this before your next encounter, or wait until performance appraisal time?

CASE STUDY: LAY OFF

You are the new office manager of a large group practice, and one of your employees is a middle-aged receptionist who has been with the practice since it started. She is a competent worker, beloved by patients and everyone who works with her. Although it was a difficult decision, the practice's current financial problems have been so great that you need to lay off at least three staff members. You have decided that the receptionist will be one of those who are let go for three reasons: her pay level is much higher than others who work the front desk; others have more computer skills than she does; and she has slowed down a bit in her work, perhaps due to some chronic health problems. Other practice leaders have reluctantly agreed with your decision about terminating the receptionist's employment, and it's now time to talk to her.

DISCUSSION QUESTIONS

1   How and where will you introduce this conversation? Will anyone else be present? Why or why not?
2   Will you tell the receptionist that this was your decision? Will you say that other practice leaders have agreed to it? Why or why not?
3   In addition to describing the practice's precarious financial situation, will you tell the receptionist about other reasons that she will be one of those to be laid off? Some of the reasons? Explain your response.
4   If the receptionist tries to get you to change your mind – noting her history at the practice, her relationships with employees and staff members, etc. – how will you let her know that this decision is not negotiable?
5   How will you handle the emotions that this discussion might bring?

CASE STUDY: ADDING INSULT TO INJURY

Mrs. Mary Lou Largely is one of the newest patients to your practice. She is 57 years old, 5'3" tall, and more than 200 pounds. The reason she left her previous health center was because her physician addressed a topic that made her very uncomfortable on each of her visits: her weight. Over time, when it was apparent that her weight was increasing rather than coming off, her doctor made comments that he thought were lighthearted, but she felt they were rude and demeaning. For example: "Come on, Mary Lou, you don't want to be a fat lady for the rest of your life, do you?" And, with a slight laugh he said, "Why haven't you gotten on the treadmill? Are you worried that you'll break it?" She left these visits humiliated and in tears, and finally decided to change physicians. Your first visit with Mrs. Largely is today.

DISCUSSION QUESTIONS

1 Assuming that you know why Mrs. Largely left the other medical practice, how would you address her weight issue with her?

2 Would you address her weight issue differently if you did not know why she left the previous practice? Please explain.

3 If Mrs. Largely did not tell you directly about her embarrassment about her weight, what would signal to you that this was something she was sensitive about?

4 What types of language would you use in addressing this issue? What words would you specifically avoid?

5 Knowing that repeated mention of Mrs. Largely's weight problems caused her to be uncomfortable in the past, what would you do or say to make these discussions easier for her to bear?

CASE STUDY: DRESS CODE

When you hired Harry Person, MD, as one of your residency program's faculty members, he had longer hair than you would have preferred, but you explained the program's rules on dress and appearance and he didn't seem to have a problem with it. Even though his job isn't in the public eye (he is now devoted to research), you are concerned because Harry's hair is even longer, he has a nose ring, and you just noticed a new tattoo on his left forearm. (The weather is excruciatingly hot and he's in short-sleeved shirts these days.) You don't want to lose Harry – he's excellent at his work and has a wonderful personality. Still, others are complaining that "Harry always gets away with things and we don't." Some say he's starting to look a little scary.

DISCUSSION QUESTIONS

1 Will you have another discussion with Dr. Person about his dress and appearance? Why or why not? Does it matter if Dr. Person is mainly doing research these days?

2 How will you address the perceptions of others that "Harry always gets away with things and we don't?" Would you tell Dr. Person's colleagues if he had been reprimanded or warned?

3 How would you approach this subject with Dr. Person? Would you mention what others have complained about?

4 What types of things would you be careful *not* to say during this conversation?

5 How would you help Dr. Person save face?

Training Tools #70

Shocking news

TYPE: Case study

ESTIMATED TRAINING TIME: 30 minutes

THEMES: Difficult conversations, emotional intelligence

OBJECTIVE:

➡ to develop skills in delivering bad news to a terminally ill patient.

MATERIALS NEEDED: A copy of the case study on the following pages for all participants

PROCEDURE:

After allowing the group a few minutes to read over the case study, ask the group the debriefing questions.

DEBRIEFING:

1 What were the problems with the way that the attending delivered the news to Mr. Headley and his family?

2 How did the attending set the tone for this discussion? What could he have done or said to have softened the blow of this news?

3 What lessons about delivering bad news were imparted to the residents by the manner and delivery of the attending's comments?

4 What was omitted from the attending's comments? What should he have said or done that he did not?

5 If you were in the attending's position, what would you have done differently?

CASE STUDY: SHOCKING NEWS

For months, Stephen Headley complained to his wife, Iris, that he was having severe headaches that seemed to be getting worse every day. When the strongest OTC medications were no longer helping, Iris took Stephen to see their primary care physician.

Along with his headaches, Stephen pointed out the stress he was experiencing from poor sales in his car business, and the need to support the Headley's two children, ages four and six. The doctor prescribed medications for Stephen's headaches, and suggested that his problems could be due to the depression that Stephen had suffered after he had to go on food stamps.

Shortly after this visit, Stephen started to stutter, and his primary care physician sent him to a neurologist. Again, Stephen mentioned his financial problems and job stress. The neurologist sent Stephen to a psychiatrist to see if the headaches and stuttering would diminish after his depression was treated.

When the stuttering and headaches became unbearable, Iris brought Stephen to the emergency room of a nearby hospital. A scan revealed that Stephen had a brain tumor, and he was admitted immediately.

The news was like a lightening bolt, but after Stephen and Iris had time to process the information, Stephen said, "At least now I know what is causing all of these symptoms and that I'm not crazy. Now we can get this taken care of. They'll operate, and life will return to normal. It has to . . . my children need me."

"So do I," Iris sobbed. "People have benign tumors all the time. You'll be fine, dear, I know it."

After a biopsy was conducted, Stephen was brought back to his room and started to awaken, with Iris at his side. Stephen's mother and sister were there too; the children were at home with a sitter.

An attending came into Stephen's private room, flanked by a team of residents. "I've just been with the surgeon and we have the results from your biopsy, Mr. Headley."

Stephen and Iris, along with Stephen's mother and sister silently began to pray that the tumor would be simple and benign. Iris even hoped that the diagnosis of a brain tumor had been a mistake in the first place. Several residents bowed their heads, somberly staring at nothing on the floor, but occasionally glancing at the family's reactions.

"It's bad news, Mr. Headley. I mean, it's really, really bad. It's the worst possible news that we could have received."

"What do you mean?" Iris asked.

"Mr. Headley, you have an anaplastic astrocytoma, Grade III. You should have had this removed six months ago and maybe we could have done something. But not only is it malignant, it's all over your brain now. It's completely inoperable. It's terminal. You and your family need to start making plans . . ."

"It-it-it's terminal?" Stephen asked, in complete disbelief. Only a few days before, he was playing catch with his six-year-old in the backyard.

"I'll say this in a way you'll understand, Mr. Headley. Think about a spider, with its arms spreading out in every direction. That's what your tumor has done. It's extended into every part of your brain. There's no way to operate. There's no way to soften what I'm telling you, and you deserve to know the truth. Like I said, this is really, really bad."

Iris began sobbing uncontrollably, unable to speak. Stephen's sister spoke up. "There has *got* to be something we can do. What about MD Anderson? Mayo? Alternative treatments?"

The attending responded with a half-laugh, half-sigh. "You can go somewhere else if it makes you feel better for trying, but there's nothing anyone can do. I've seen some brain tumors this bad in which the patient has lived for six months, so you might make it six months too, but in your case I seriously doubt it. I always tell people, 'hope for the best and expect the worst.' But your tumor is so bad it's time for you to make plans and get your house in order."

As he edged toward the door, the attending repeated, "It's too bad you didn't take care of this before, Mr. Headley. Six months ago we might have been able to do something." The attending and residents left the room, and the three women hugged Stephen, a flood of tears rolling down their cheeks. Iris slunk to the floor as she saw her husband begin to curl into a fetal position.

Six role-play
exercises with
two players and an
observer

Training Tools #71–6

Difficult conversations – role-play exercises

TYPE: Role play

ESTIMATED TRAINING TIME: 90 minutes (three cases)

THEME: Difficult conversations

OBJECTIVE:

➡ to hone skills in conducting difficult conversations in a variety of situations.

MATERIALS NEEDED: Copies of two character roles and the observer sheet for each triad for the three exercises you select

PROCEDURE:

Divide participants into groups of three. For each case, give two persons in each triad a different character role and the other the observer sheet. Note that the role of observer should be alternated so that each person has a chance to serve in that role, which requires analyzing the interaction and suggesting improvements immediately after the scene.

Select three of the following exercises to role play during the 90-minute time frame:

➡ **Consoling thoughts** – Colleagues need a grieving co-worker to step up to the plate.

➡ **A malignant situation** – Tell a patient that his cancer has returned.

➡ **It's hard to say** – Talk to a patient who is embarrassed to ask for contraceptives.

➡ **Getting ahead** – Tell an argumentative doctor that he won't receive a promotion.

➡ **The nose knows** – Tell a hospital volunteer that he has body odor.

➡ **Cloud of suspicion** – Express suspicions that a resident is high from marijuana.

To complete all three exercises, suggest that each group spend approximately 15 minutes or so for each role play, using the remaining time to discuss the observer's observations and recommendations.

DEBRIEFING:

As you reconvene the entire group, ask for a reporter from each triad to report on the key points from their discussion. During this discussion, ask how the strategies differed from one type of difficult conversation to another.

ROLE PLAY: CONSOLING THOUGHTS
CONFIDENTIAL INSTRUCTIONS

Nursing Supervisor

One of your employees, Nora Nightengale, RN, is returning to work after two weeks' absence to attend her father's funeral and tie up loose ends at her family's home. Nora's father, who was 88 years old, suffered from Alzheimer's disease. During the last few months, you have tried to be as compassionate as possible, giving Nora extra days off so that she could assist other family members with caregiver responsibilities. When she did come to work, she often appeared tired and distracted; in fact, several colleagues noticed a major decrease in her productivity. While you are quite sorry about her loss, you would like Nora to start working at full capacity as soon as possible. The two people who have been covering for Nora are both pregnant – one is in her last trimester – and they are particularly anxious for Nora to start carrying her share of the workload.

ROLE PLAY: CONSOLING THOUGHTS
CONFIDENTIAL INSTRUCTIONS

Nora Nightengale, RN

You are Nora Nightengale, RN, and you have just returned from a week at your family's home to attend your father's funeral. He was 88 years old and suffered from Alzheimer's disease, and for the last six months you took extra time off work to assist your family in his care. As a nurse, your family depended on you more than anyone else. You are exhausted – physically as well as emotionally. While your father's passing was not unexpected, you have been so busy attending to details that you don't feel that you've had sufficient time to grieve. Now that you are back at work, you worry that your colleagues will demand more of you than you are able to give. You know that you haven't been working up to speed for several months, but feel more drained now than ever.

ROLE PLAY: CONSOLING THOUGHTS

Questions for Observer

1. How did the supervisor acknowledge Nora's loss?
2. Did the supervisor address the organization's needs during this conversation? If so, was that done with sensitivity for Nora's emotional state?
3. Did the supervisor offer help and support? How?
4. Did the supervisor say anything inappropriate, such as "It was a blessing; you must be relieved," or "Aren't you over it yet?"
5. What did the supervisor do especially well during this role play?
6. What improvements in verbal or nonverbal behaviors would you suggest?

ROLE PLAY: A MALIGNANT SITUATION
CONFIDENTIAL INSTRUCTIONS

Primary Care Physician

You are Tom Jefferson, MD, and you'll soon be seeing one of your patients, Mr. Jon Adams, age 43. You are not looking forward to this visit. It has been nearly four and a half years since Mr. Adams had lung cancer surgery, and he's been in excellent spirits, thinking that he was not far from his five-year remission mark. You've just learned from the lab that Mr. Adams' cancer has recurred, and there is evidence that it may have metastasized. While you will suggest several treatment options, you know that this news will be especially devastating since both of Mr. Adams' parents and two grandparents passed away from various types of cancer before age 60. Mr. Adams and his wife have three small children, and Mrs. Adams depends on her husband a great deal, especially now that she has been diagnosed with fibromyalgia.

ROLE PLAY: A MALIGNANT SITUATION
CONFIDENTIAL INSTRUCTIONS

Jon Adams, Patient

You are Mr. Jon Adams, age 43. You're looking forward to today's office visit with your primary care physician, Dr. Tom Jefferson. It's been more than four years since your lung cancer surgery, and you aren't far from reaching five years of remission — at which point you plan to take your wife and three children to your favorite resort for a celebration. Your wife, who has recently been diagnosed with fibromyalgia, believes that the salt water will do wonders for her pain. If the doctor tells you good news today about your most recent test, you'll go ahead and make your family's plane reservations.

If you did hear bad news you would be so shocked you could barely speak. In that case, the doctor will have to carry the ball on this interaction.

ROLE PLAY: A MALIGNANT SITUATION

Questions for Observer

1   How did Dr. Jefferson break the news to Mr. Adams? Did he preface his remarks, or get right to the point? Knowing Mr. Adams' background and current circumstances, which approach is preferable?

2   What was the sequence of Dr. Jefferson's discussion? Did he follow the bad news with positive statements about treatment options? Were the positive comments realistic?

3   Did Dr. Jefferson give the news all at once, or in parts? Did the patient send cues about how much information to give or what direction the conversation should take?

4   Did Dr. Jefferson ask if any family members could be there for support, either to hear the news, take him home, or both?

5   How did Dr. Jefferson deal with Mr. Adams' reaction? How did he address Mr. Adams' likely impression that, for him, this news was tantamount to a death sentence?

6   Was there too much talking? Were Dr. Jefferson and Mr. Adams able to share a quiet moment in sorrow?

ROLE PLAY: IT'S HARD TO SAY
CONFIDENTIAL INSTRUCTIONS

Physician

You are about to see a patient for the third time: a high school student, Lisa Looper, age 14. In previous visits for her asthma, it has occurred to you that Lisa might be sexually active. You raised the question as skillfully as you could; she seemed extremely reticent to talk with you about it. She refuses a gynecological exam, but tells you that she does not see another doctor for these services, and acts extremely nervous when you ask such questions. She has not listed contraceptives on her medical history forms. You have the distinct impression that there's something she'd like to ask or discuss, but can't find the courage.

She's coming back for an asthma-related visit today, but you would like to open the door to a full discussion with Lisa about what's going on.

Training Tool #73

ROLE PLAY: IT'S HARD TO SAY
CONFIDENTIAL INSTRUCTIONS

Lisa Looper, Patient

You are Lisa Looper, a 14-year-old high school student from a very conservative family. While you like your new physician, you are surprised about the questions that were asked during your previous three visits to the doctor regarding your sexual behavior. You acted very reluctant to talk about such things, but you know it was apparent that you were nervous the last time your doctor asked about it, so you're pretty certain the subject will come up again.

The truth is, you have had sexual relations with a boy at school several times so far. You're not terribly worried about getting pregnant – after all, Todd usually remembers to buy condoms – but if you ever got the nerve, you'd like to ask about some contraceptives that a friend is taking. But whenever you think of asking, you talk yourself out of it. Your mother and father have no idea that you have been having sex already and they would be extremely disappointed in you. You know they'd make you go talk to your minister, and they'd most likely ground you for so long that you'd never get to see Todd again.

Your office visit today is about your asthma again. Whether or not you break your silence about this "sex issue" depends on how the doctor talks about it. Before you breathe a word of this, you really want to be sure that your mother and father don't find out.

ROLE PLAY: IT'S HARD TO SAY

Questions for Observer

1 How might the doctor have known that the patient had questions but was embarrassed to ask?

2 How did the doctor help Lisa open up about this issue? What verbal, nonverbal, and listening techniques were used?

3 Did the doctor ask questions to uncover Lisa's misperceptions about birth control?

4 Did the doctor go beyond this issue by making efforts to build a more trusting relationship overall?

5 How did the doctor's communication come across to Lisa?

6 If the conversation got that far, how did the doctor handle the issue of confidentiality?

ROLE PLAY: GETTING AHEAD
CONFIDENTIAL INSTRUCTIONS

Barry White, MD, Residency Director

You are Barry White, MD, director of a large family medicine residency program. Because your associate director decided to accept a position in another State, you must select her successor. After careful thought, you've decided to hire Dr. Lana Lane for this position. Even though Dr. Lane has never worked at your hospital before, you worked with her at another medical center several years ago and remain impressed with her excellent administrative skills and professional judgment.

Today, you will have to tell Dr. Jimmy Molson that he did not get the job, even though you realize he expects it. Although you have no complaints about Dr. Molson's work as a faculty member for the past six years, you find him "high maintenance" because he tends to be argumentative. By hiring Dr. Lane, you believe you'll have a better chance for teamwork at the top — essential for a smooth-running program.

ROLE PLAY: GETTING AHEAD
CONFIDENTIAL INSTRUCTIONS

Jimmy Molson, MD, Faculty Member

You are Dr. Jimmy Molson, a faculty member at a large family medicine residency program. You are looking forward to today's meeting with Dr. Barry White, the program director, because you'll find out if you've been selected as the new associate director.

You believe you have an excellent chance. You've received excellent performance evaluations for the past six years, and the director's only complaint has been that you're somewhat argumentative. You disagree, seeing yourself as unafraid to introduce new ideas that elevate the quality of decision making. If the director doesn't select you – or if he brings in someone from the outside – you'll be furious.

ROLE PLAY: GETTING AHEAD

Questions for Observer

1   How did Dr. White present this news to Dr. Molson? Did he focus on why he selected Dr. Lane, why Dr. Molson didn't get the job, or both? Did he do this in a way that will avoid future relationship problems between Drs. Lane and Molson?

2   What emotions and identity issues were underlying the discussion? Were these issues openly addressed? If so, did it help or hinder the interaction?

3   What efforts were made to help Dr. Molson save face? Why is that important?

4   What did Dr. White do, if anything, to avert new layers of conflict over a decision he'd already made?

5   What should both parties have done differently?

ROLE PLAY: THE NOSE KNOWS
CONFIDENTIAL INSTRUCTIONS

Hospital Volunteer Coordinator

OD Ferris is a 72-year-old man who lost his wife to heart disease a few years ago and was quite depressed and lonely until he began working at your hospital as a volunteer. As the hospital volunteer coordinator, you are Mr. Ferris' supervisor. You think Mr. Ferris is surely one of the kindest, most sensitive souls you've ever met. When he is embarrassed — which is frequent, as sensitive as he is — his cheeks turns a bright shade of red that makes everyone laugh.

Ever since Mr. Ferris began working as a volunteer 10 months ago, you assigned him to usher visitors to the radiology lab. Your hospital is extremely large and has many twists and turns, and the hallways aren't always easy to navigate. Mr. Ferris has loved this job because he gets to exercise and, even better, he gets to talk to patients, family members, and visitors during his walks.

During the past few weeks, several visitors asked for assistance in finding the radiology department, but when Mr. Ferris came to assist them, they thanked him but said they changed their minds, noting that they could find radiology themselves. You also noticed that Mr. Ferris is by himself more frequently rather than talking to the other volunteers like he used to.

You decided to talk to Mr. Ferris to see if you could figure out what the problem might be. As soon as you walked up to him, you almost passed out from the smell, which seemed something like spoiled fish. You didn't say anything to him at the time, but you decided that you must say something to him for the sake of his coworkers, the visitors, and Mr. Ferris himself.

ROLE PLAY: THE NOSE KNOWS
CONFIDENTIAL INSTRUCTIONS

OD Ferris, Hospital Volunteer

You are OD Ferris, a 72-year-old man who lost his wife to heart disease a few years ago. You were quite depressed and lonely after your wife passed away, but every-thing changed after you became a volunteer at your local hospital. It is your reason for getting up in the morning!

You think the people you work with are just wonderful (though you can't figure out why they don't seem to be talking to you as much as they used to), and you especially like your supervisor, the volunteer coordinator (even though you usually only see the coordinator when something goes wrong). Thankfully, most things that do go wrong aren't because of anything you've done. You don't take criticism well, and you are extremely sensitive. Sometimes people laugh when they see how red your face gets when you're embarrassed!

Ever since you began volunteering at the hospital, you've been assigned to usher visitors to the radiology lab. The hospital is extremely large and has many twists and turns, and the hallways aren't always easy to navigate. How you love this job! Not only do you get to exercise, you also get to talk to patients, family members, and visitors during your walks.

However, during the past few weeks you've tried to help several visitors find the radiology department, but they thanked you and said they didn't need your help after all. You don't understand; your personality hasn't changed a bit! And because the other volunteers haven't been talking to you as much, you've been keeping to yourself.

Oh no, here comes the volunteer coordinator. You hope you didn't do anything wrong. You hate to be criticized. Your dearly departed wife used to do that.

ROLE PLAY: THE NOSE KNOWS

Questions for Observer

1 How did the supervisor tell Mr. Ferris about his body odor?

2 Was the language appropriate? If not, was the choice of words so diplomatic that the message was obscured? Or was the message so direct that it came across as blaming and hurtful?

3 Were efforts made to help Mr. Ferris maintain his dignity? To be less embarrassed?

4 What nonverbal behaviors help to convey the message as intended?

5 What solutions were suggested?

6 Did the conversation end on a good note?

ROLE PLAY: CLOUD OF SUSPICION
CONFIDENTIAL INSTRUCTIONS

Residency Director

You've asked one of the residents in your program to see you in your office today. What you plan to discuss will be difficult, because it's about your suspicion that this resident is high on marijuana or some other substance. Several observations and rumors about this resident have led to your misgivings; for example:

▶ loud talking, sometimes slurred, with intermittent bursts of laughter;

▶ drooping eyes – practically shut – making you think that sometimes the resident is about to keel over;

▶ lack of concentration;

▶ frequent forgetfulness;

▶ comments from other residents who have wondered if this resident was "high."

You don't have any proof, just speculation, but the rumors you've heard from the chief resident and other residents about this resident's possible drug use have been increasing, and you've wondered if they are aware of specifics that they're not telling you about. As far as you know, this resident has still been performing quite well, and you were quite impressed with how the resident managed a patient with diabetes. You haven't told the resident yet, but you just received a letter from the patient to tell you how much she appreciated all that the resident did for her.

You are concerned enough about this situation that that you feel the need to find out for yourself what's going on. If necessary, you have thought about asking the resident to submit to a drug test.

ROLE PLAY: CLOUD OF SUSPICION
CONFIDENTIAL INSTRUCTIONS

Resident

You wonder why the residency program director has asked to see you today. Maybe it's to tell you what a great job you did managing a patient's diabetes – or maybe you're in trouble for something. You can't imagine what, though.

Sure, you admit that you've slowed down quite a bit lately. You haven't been sleeping well, and you suspect that's why it's been hard to maintain your concentration at times and why you've been forgetting things that you normally remember. It's also possibly why you look in the mirror and wonder who you're looking at; your eyes are practically at half-mast.

You don't want your lack of sleep to be an issue at your residency, so you try to compensate for that by showing your great personality to others. You enjoy socializing with your colleagues, and there are two residents that you have so much fun with that people can hear your peals of laughter all the way down the hall. Of course, they mainly hear you, because you have a naturally loud voice.

Although you aren't quite certain why the residency director wants to see you, you wonder if it is due to comments by other residents who jokingly asked if you were smoking marijuana or taking other kinds of drugs. You shrugged off these comments in the past – even when the chief resident said that your denials were not very convincing. You would be much more upset and quite embarrassed if the residency director asked you about this. You would agree to take a drug test, but you'd be highly insulted if the residency director didn't take you at your word.

ROLE PLAY: CLOUD OF SUSPICION

Questions for Observer

1 Was it justifiable for the director to voice suspicions about the resident?

2 Was the director questioning the resident objectively and with concern, or was it accusatory?

3 How could the resident have explained that drugs were not an issue without seeming overly defensive?

4 Did the director find out about the resident's sleeping problem? If so, how was that addressed?

5 If the resident felt hurt about the subject of the conversation, how did the director handle that?

6 Did the residency director ask the resident to take a drug test? If so, was that appropriate? Or should the resident have been taken at his/her word?

Communicating in crisis situations

The potential for crises

TYPE: Introductory discussion

ESTIMATED TRAINING TIME: 15 minutes

THEME: Communicating in crisis situations

OBJECTIVES:
➡ to identify the types of crises, disasters, and emergencies that could occur;
➡ to understand the need for readiness.

MATERIALS NEEDED: Flip chart

PROCEDURE:
To introduce the topic, "Communicating in Crisis Situations," ask participants, "What potential types of crisis situations could we encounter in our geographic area? What types might we encounter in our facility?" Ask for specific examples of potential crises within these categories and display the group's responses on a flip chart.

After the list is complete, ask the group to identify the audiences to whom they must communicate for each type of crisis. Depending on the type of health care organization, potential audiences may include the medical staff, nursing staff, office workers, patients, administration, board members, community groups, and the media.

DEBRIEFING:
Use this discussion to point out the need for emergency planning, noting that disasters require not only clinical expertise but attention to a myriad of details and a plan for communicating essential information to various groups. Then consider:
1 What messages need to be conveyed to each audience for each type of crisis?
2 What are the best methods of conveying those messages?
3 How do the messages and methods differ for each type of crisis or audience type?

The need to
address glitches
in organizational
communication
before a crisis
occurs

Training Tool #78

From bad to worse

TYPE: Introductory discussion

ESTIMATED TRAINING TIME: 15 minutes

THEME: Communicating in crisis situations

OBJECTIVE:

➡ to understand that existing communication glitches in an organization often worsen during a crisis – a time when the highest level of effective communication is needed most.

MATERIALS NEEDED: Flip chart

PROCEDURE:

Point out that existing communication problems in an organization are likely to worsen when a crisis strikes. Then ask the following questions.

DEBRIEFING:

1 What are some possible reasons that this would be true? Would emotionalism, being in a rush, or other factors come into play?

2 What communication channels in our organization/facility do you think would be most likely to break down during a crisis situation? (Point out that communication channels are the methods of communicating from one party to another, e.g. between providers, between departments, with administrative personnel, with community groups, the media, etc.)

3 Which existing communication problems in our organization do we most need to correct so that we can coordinate timely and effective responses to emergencies and crisis situations?

If participants become stuck when trying to think of the various types of communication problems, ask them to evaluate the quality of communication in these categories: general communication; team communication; leadership/management communication; conflict management; meetings; decision making; lateral communication; and external communication.

Training Tool #79

Identifying the risk
factors for a crisis in
a hospital

Signal detection

TYPE: Introductory discussion

ESTIMATED TRAINING TIME: 30 minutes

THEME: Communicating in crisis situations

OBJECTIVES:
- to identify risk factors for a potential crisis in a hospital setting;
- to determine how those factors should influence plans for essential types of communication.

MATERIALS NEEDED: Flip chart

PROCEDURE:

Ask participants to imagine that they are at a hospital that is now opening a new birthing facility. They are members of a committee that will develop plans for the security of the neonatal nursery in order to protect against the unlikely possibility that newborns would be kidnapped.

Draw two columns on the flipchart, and list the following headings at the top of each: Equipment and Education. Then ask the group the following questions and write their responses in the appropriate columns:

- What *equipment* would be needed to ensure safety? (Possible answers are video cameras, alarm devices, indicators to show which exit doors had been open, an electronic ID tag tied to the baby's ankle, etc.)
- Which parties would you need to *educate* about security risks? (Nursery staff and parents)
   - What would you need to educate **nursery staff** to do? (Wear photo ID badges unique to the hospital; keep the infant in sight by a parent or nursery staff member at all times; forbid anyone to take an infant anywhere without identification; only give information to people you know and trust; study typical abduction scenarios to know what to look out for; etc.)
   - What would you need to educate **parents** to do? (Know the hospital's security procedures; know the doctors and nurses; keep the bassinet next to you and away from the door; know when tests are scheduled; etc.)

DEBRIEFING:

After developing the lists, ask these questions:

1   What types of communication would be necessary within the hospital about the nursery's security equipment?

2   What is the best way to provide training to orient new nursery staff members about security precautions? What is the best way to ensure communication about security matters from one shift to another?

3   Who should communicate with parents about security within the birthing center? How can you do this with sensitivity so that parents are not unnecessarily fearful, especially while they might be in a sensitive, emotional state?

4   What types of communication between nursery staff and parents are important throughout the family's time spent in the birthing facility?

Case studies in crisis communication

TYPE: Case studies (two cases)

ESTIMATED TRAINING TIME: 60 minutes

THEME: Communicating in crisis situations

OBJECTIVES:
➡ to identify ways to handle small-scale crises involving only a few people or a community;
➡ to demonstrate that crisis situations often entail both internal and external communication issues.

MATERIALS NEEDED: A copy of two selected cases for all participants

PROCEDURE:
Break the group into teams of four or five persons, distribute two case studies, and note that each team should allow around 15 minutes to discuss each of the two cases. (You can review more cases if time allows.) Your options are as follows:
➡ **Heard it through the grapevine** – Rumors run wild about a possible downsizing.
➡ **Inevitable outcome** – A patient's death leaves questions of a medication overdose.
➡ **A scary world** – An anonymous caller reports anthrax contamination through the mail.
➡ **Oh, rats!** – Word gets out about rodent infestation at a hospital.

Note that one person from each group will be asked to report to the group as a whole on the team's responses to the questions that appear after each scenario.

CASE STUDY: HEARD IT THROUGH THE GRAPEVINE

Established 20 years ago, the Supreme Medical Group is now the largest multi-specialty group practice in your county. The expansion of the practice started about 10 years ago, when a major automobile manufacturing plant in the area expanded its operations. To care for the area's burgeoning population, the practice today has 30 people: 8 physicians, 7 nurses, 6 reception staff, and 9 administrative staff. Many have been at the practice from the beginning.

Because the automobile plant manufactured large cars, trucks, and SUVs, the demand for its products diminished considerably when gas prices increased. With major financial problems, the plant completely closed its truck and SUV production areas, and nearly 2000 people have been laid off from their jobs during the past year. Many have since moved out of town.

Recently, a distraught receptionist at Supreme Medical Group told a nurse about a rumor floating around town that four of the eight doctors would be leaving – meaning, of course, that numerous other employees would lose their jobs. Within the day, everyone who worked at the practice had heard the rumor.

Fearful of panicking everyone who works at the practice about possible job losses, the physicians assembled into a conference room to decide what to do. They acknowledge to one another that it is indeed possible that some of them would leave if the practice didn't perk up, even though no one had decided to leave as of yet.

DISCUSSION QUESTIONS

1 What could have been done to avoid this situation?
2 Should the doctors address the concerns of those who work at the practice? Or should they simply dismiss the rumor as malicious gossip?
3 What is the potential harm to the practice if patients hear the rumor?
4 Since the rumor began in the community, should practice leaders address the rumor with the media? Or should they wait until something has been decided?

CASE STUDY: INEVITABLE OUTCOME

Mrs. Leona Hambly has had emphysema for at least 10 years, but her condition worsened tremendously during the past year. After Leona's husband, Harry, died a few years ago, their daughter, Harriet, began to notice during weekly visits that her mother had lost more weight, but this didn't seem to be adding to the problem.

Last week, while looking out one of the windows of her luxurious penthouse overlooking the city, Mrs. Hambly began to feel even more fatigued and short-of-breath than usual. She called Harriet immediately, but couldn't gather the strength to answer the door when Harriet arrived. After Harriet got the doorman to break in with the master key, she saw her mother's weakened condition and immediately called an ambulance.

Mrs. Hambly was taken to the emergency room at Amazing Grace Hospital, and Harriet arrived shortly thereafter. Harriet watched the commotion as a team of hospital personnel busily swarmed around her mother, conducting tests and giving her an injection. To Harriet's utter shock, Mrs. Hambly was soon pronounced dead. In disbelief, Harriet couldn't understand what had happened; her mother had bounced back from far worse episodes than this one numerous times before.

More than an hour later, with Harriet still grieving at her mother's bedside, one of the physicians called Harriet aside and told her that Mrs. Hambly passed away after being given a high dose of steroids and albuterol. A nurse who accompanied the doctor was trying to soothe Harriet when she said, "Harriet, your mother was so sick. If she didn't die today, she would have died soon anyway." The physician nodded in agreement.

Harriet couldn't believe her ears. She had just learned that her mother passed away, and the way she interpreted what was said, it seemed like her death was caused by a drug overdose! But what kept replaying in Harriet's mind was the nurse saying, "She would have died soon anyway." Harriet was furious with the audaciousness of that comment.

Harriett decided to file suit against the hospital. She also contacted a reporter at the local newspaper and said, "Is your pen ready? I have your next big story."

DISCUSSION QUESTIONS

1 Should the physician have explained more about the use of steroids and albuterol? What could have been said to Harriet so that she would realize that there wasn't a direct relationship between the medications and her mother's death?

2 After telling Harriet that her mother had died after being given the two medications,

could anything have been done or said to have caused Harriet not to file a lawsuit against the hospital?

3 What were the problems with what the nurse said to Harriet?
4 What sympathy or comfort was offered to Harriet?
5 Which parties from the hospital should speak with the newspaper? What information should be conveyed?

CASE STUDY: A SCARY WORLD

Stephanie Steddy, a switchboard operator at Majestic Medical Center was stunned when she received an anonymous phone call stating that an anthrax-contaminated letter had been mailed to the medical center. She asked the caller to stay on the line while she called someone for help, but the caller hung up.

Stephanie wasn't sure what to do. Should she call her supervisor first? Should she call the hospital administrator? Or should she call the mail room and tell them not to open anything?

She decided to call the hospital administrator, Phil Frenzy, but was told that he was in a meeting. "Get him on the phone NOW! It's an emergency!" Stephanie urged. Mr. Frenzy's assistant, Betty Blabbit, asked about the nature of the emergency. When Stephanie said that she'd prefer to tell the administrator personally, Betty said, "Sorry, but if I'm going to pull Mr. Frenzy out of an important meeting, I need to know what this is about."

Reluctantly, Stephanie told Betty about the call. "You were right to tell me," Betty said. "I'll get Mr. Frenzy right away."

As Betty ran to the conference room where Mr. Frenzy was meeting, two nurses were talking in the hallway. "Where's the fire?" one said. "Slow down, Betty; you could have knocked us over!"

"It's not a fire," Betty replied frantically. "It's worse. We have an anthrax threat and I've got to get Phil out of his meeting right away!" Nearby, a patient's family heard the exchange and began to panic.

Just as all of this was happening, a local television station received an anonymous call about the contaminated letter that was sent to Majestic Medical Center.

DISCUSSION QUESTIONS

1 Was Stephanie justified in revealing the problem to Betty Blabbit? Why or why not?

2 Did Stephanie make the best choice by deciding to contact the hospital administrator first? Please explain.

3 Does it matter how this matter is handled if the threat is a hoax or if the contamination is real?

4 What can the administrator or any other party do to contain the panic that is likely to ensue?

5 Which individuals or groups should the administrator contact first to address this threat?

6 How should the medical center deal with the media?

7 What other issues or problems might be involved?

8 How would the actions differ if this were a bomb threat instead?

CASE STUDY: OH, RATS!

As soon as the kitchen staff at Mayberry Rehabilitation Center noticed a gnawed hole in one of the walls, they told administrative leaders that they suspected a rodent problem. They were right. Just as Andy Saylor, the executive director, was about to take action, a large rat was seen scampering down the hall.

Andy called exterminators to take care of the problem. Bait and traps were placed strategically throughout the kitchen and the contractors conducted a deep clean of the kitchen, pantry, and dining room with chemicals and pesticides. Arrangements were made to have food brought in from a local caterer while the kitchen was temporarily closed.

Amidst these efforts, Helen Strump, a physical therapist, ran to Andy's office in tears.

"I cannot believe there are rats here," Helen said. "We have patients here with post-surgical and traumatic injuries; some can't get around without assistance and some can't move. Who knows what diseases these rats are carrying?"

Andy pointed out that he was handling the problem as best he could. He explained that the problem started with a new system in the kitchen to compost waste and that the problem had now been addressed. In fact, he pointed out, he was just about to send a notice to the entire staff to explain that the problem was now under control.

"You're kidding," Helen said. "You've only been addressing the problem in the kitchen and dining hall, but I just saw droppings on the third floor!"

"Helen, I urge you not to make matters worse," Andy urged. "Please don't tell others what you saw. I don't believe that was you saw were droppings – it had to be something else – but in any case, I'll look into it. Don't forget that our hospital has recently been rated as 'excellent' for cleanliness, and we care about nothing more than our patients' safety. That goes for the staff, too, so I'd really appreciate you keeping this to yourself. You don't want us to be closed down, do you?"

DISCUSSION QUESTIONS

1   Was Andy justified in asking Helen to keep silent about the possibility of additional evidence of the problem? Why or why not? Was it a factor that Andy had not checked out Helen's claim yet?

2   What should Andy say to calm the persons that Helen most likely already told about what she saw?

3   What, if anything, should be communicated to the patients and their families who obviously notice that the kitchen has been closed?

4   Should Helen notify the local public health department if Andy does not?

5 What messages should be conveyed to the media? Should the media be contacted even if they don't contact the hospital for a statement first?

6 What other types of damage control can the rehabilitation center do in order to avoid being perceived by the community as unclean or dangerous?

Crisis response

TYPE: Role play

ESTIMATED TRAINING TIME: 60 minutes

THEME: Communicating in crisis situations

OBJECTIVE:

➡ to know the importance of following the nine steps of crisis response when an event occurs.

MATERIALS NEEDED: Copies of the case study on the following page for all participants

For teaching this session, it will help to obtain a copy of *Crisis and Emergency Risk Communication*. (*See* Further Reading list under "Communicating in Crisis Situations.")

PROCEDURE:

In a brief lecture, identify the nine steps of crisis response recommended by the Centers for Disease Control and Prevention.

1 Verify information
2 Conduct notifications
3 Conduct crisis assessment (activate crisis plan)
4 Organize assignments (organizational issues, partner involvement)
5 Prepare information and obtain approvals
6 Release information to media, public, and partners through arranged channels
7 Obtain feedback and conduct crisis evaluation
8 Conduct public education
9 Monitor events

(See the abovementioned book for more detail on each step.)

Ask participants to form small groups and note that they will each play the role of a hospital leader. You can let the groups designate their own roles (e.g. administrator, associate administrator, medical director, nursing director, chief financial operator, director of infectious disease control, etc.) Tell participants they will have 40 minutes to discuss how they will respond to this crisis described in the case study using the nine-step process.

ROLE PLAY: CRISIS RESPONSE

It seemed to be a typical childhood accident. Timmy Partin, age seven, was playing with his dog, Sassie, throwing a Frisbee and running in the woods behind the house where he lived with his mother Ruth and father Paul. Ruth and Paul heard the dog barking loudly and ran outside to see if there was a problem. They soon discovered Timmy on the ground, writhing in pain and crying, "My leg! My leg!"

Ruth and Paul rushed Timmy to the nearest hospital where it was found that he had broken his right leg in several places. Surgery was immediately scheduled, and Timmy's parents took turns staying overnight with him in the hospital for the next few days. Shortly thereafter, Timmy's leg became red, swollen, and painful from numerous abscesses with a great deal of pus. A test for staphylococcus came back positive.

Days later, eight more patients developed symptoms of a staph infection, and there are signs that some of these infections are resistant to antibiotics.

You and other hospital leaders are now meeting to discuss what steps to take to deal with this crisis. You plan to follow the nine steps of crisis response recommended by the Centers for Disease Control and Prevention. What will you and other leaders recommend for each step?

1 Verify information
2 Conduct notifications
3 Conduct crisis assessment (activate crisis plan)
4 Organize assignments (organizational issues, partner involvement)
5 Prepare information and obtain approvals
6 Release information to media, public, and partners through arranged channels
7 Obtain feedback and conduct crisis evaluation
8 Conduct public education
9 Monitor events

Dealing with organizational change

My personal experience with change

TYPE: Worksheet

ESTIMATED TRAINING TIME: 15 minutes

THEME: Organizational change

OBJECTIVE:

➡ to realize that many types of change are possible in health care settings, with some easier to adapt to than others.

MATERIALS NEEDED: A copy of the worksheet on the following page for all participants

PROCEDURE:

Distribute a copy of the worksheet to all participants and give them a few minutes to fill it out.

DEBRIEFING:

1 In the first section of the worksheet, how did each of you describe change that occurs in association with your work? How many said "exhilarating"? (Expect laughter!)
2 Which types of changes were the most difficult to adapt to? Which were the least difficult? Why?
3 Considering how various types of changes were introduced and managed, what are some examples of things that were done that made the transition process easier on you and your coworkers?
4 What would help you to better deal with future organizational changes? Please explain.

Worksheet

MY PERSONAL EXPERIENCE WITH CHANGE
I define change in connection with my work as:

_____

_____

_____

During the past two years, I have experienced the following changes:

____ Reorganization of my department

____ New reporting relationships

____ Modifications in services

____ New technology

____ Reduction in work force

____ New/different responsibilities

____ Major policy revisions

____ New goals or projects

____ Centralization

____ De-centralization

____ New work standards

____ Transfer to a new work group

____ Changes in the hours of work

____ Relocation of the office

____ Revision of the incentive program

____ Introduction of a new performance appraisal system

____ Changes in pay structure

____ Merger with another organization

Add your own:

_____

_____

_____

Changes in an interdependent system

TYPE: Introductory discussion

ESTIMATED TRAINING TIME: 30 minutes

THEME: Organizational change

OBJECTIVES:

➡ to understand that a change initiated in one area or department is likely to have an impact upon others or require their participation;

➡ to underscore the importance of effective communication with all persons, areas, and departments affected by a change.

MATERIALS NEEDED: Flip chart

PROCEDURE:

Provide a brief lecture about the interdependent nature of health care, e.g. the need for teamwork among various professions and disciplines and the interactions that are necessary between one unit or department and another, as well as with other organizations and agencies. Point out that when we initiate a change in an interdependent organization, we must take into account which other groups or individuals are likely to be affected; after all, the change may require them to take action or do something differently.

Give the group the following examples and ask, "Which parties are likely to be impacted by each of the following changes"?

➡ You are the office manager at a private practice and have developed a new patient appointment method.

➡ You've decided to add a nutritionist to your staff for the first time.

➡ You are a family nurse practitioner and you've just decided it's time to retire.

DEBRIEFING:

1 Did you notice that the changes we've discussed involve communication with numerous parties, not just one or two?

2 What would happen if you didn't communicate with everyone that needed to be informed or educated?

3 What different types of information would need to be conveyed to the different parties in these situations?

Identifying what the
organization can do
to help personnel
adjust to multiple
changes

Training Tool #87

An association in turmoil

TYPE: Case study

ESTIMATED TRAINING TIME: 30 minutes

THEMES: Organizational change, conflict management

OBJECTIVES:

➡ to realize the complexities of dealing with numerous types of changes simultaneously;

➡ to identify ways to assist personnel in their efforts to adapt to multiple simultaneous changes.

MATERIALS NEEDED: A copy of the case study on the following page for all participants

PROCEDURE:

Distribute the case study and ask participants to discuss it in small groups. Then bring the group back together and ask the following questions.

DEBRIEFING:

1 Would you even need to address the association's changes that people feel are essential? Why or why not?

2 Would you do anything differently to help people deal with negative changes (e.g. budget reductions) than you would to help them deal with positive changes (e.g. adding new areas of emphasis)? If so, what?

3 Would it be best to develop strategies to help personnel adapt to one change at a time – or all at once?

4 Which of the changes are likely to cause the greatest resistance? The least resistance?

5 What will you recommend for reducing tensions in each of the remaining offices?

6 What strategies would be most effective for helping personnel adjust to these changes? Approximately how long do you estimate that this process will take?

CASE STUDY: AN ASSOCIATION IN TURMOIL

You are a leader in an association that is dedicated to improving the quality and accessibility of health care for communities within the State through a system of community-academic partnerships. The central purposes of your association are to recruit, educate, and retain primary health providers.

Although the association has been running smoothly for years, there is a feeling of unsettlement among some staff members and others as a result of several significant changes in the association during the past year. Changes include: State budget reductions (which are causing the association to downsize the number of its statewide field offices from seven to four); new areas of emphasis (a good thing!); and the need to develop a new technology plan for the association's operating system. Another change involves the recent turnover of personnel. Several key staff members have left, and new staff members have been hired – either as replacements or to assume newly created positions. As a result, many veteran staff members of the association are now working with people they don't yet know.

While most leaders of the association and a growing number of staff members believe that the changes were essential, you want to do something to facilitate people's adaptation to these changes and reduce the lingering tensions. You will now meet with several colleagues – faculty, site directors, and site personnel – to brainstorm on things that the association might do.

When software is hard

TYPE: Case study

ESTIMATED TRAINING TIME: 30 minutes

THEMES: Organizational change, conflict management

OBJECTIVE:

➡ to identify ways to deal with change when problems develop during implementation.

MATERIALS NEEDED: A copy of the case study on the next page for all participants

PROCEDURE:

After a brief overview about organizational change, give the group a few minutes to read the role play and ask the following questions.

DEBRIEFING:

1 What should be on the agenda for the all-staff meeting about the problems that some have experienced with the EMR?

2 How can those who are happy with the EMR system be most helpful to others?

3 Should Dr. Rankle be excused from using some of the core features of the EMR, even though he agreed to use these features when this came up a year ago? What would be the effect on his colleagues who *are* using all the core features? Does it matter that Dr. Rankle has decided to retire in a year?

4 If Darla expresses her concerns at the meeting – and if it's not yet certain whether any medical records technicians will be laid off – is there anything that could be said to assuage her fears?

5 What are the options for helping medical records technicians to facilitate their learning curve?

6 How could some, if not most, of these problems have been avoided?

CASE STUDY: WHEN SOFTWARE IS HARD

You've recently installed a new Electronic Medical Record (EMR) system in your practice and so far, the reviews have been mixed.

- Dr. Zelda Zeal, who has been the key champion for the EMR within your practice, has been raving about the increased efficiencies. "I've been able to go home from work about an hour earlier – all because of the EMR!" Dr. Zeal exclaimed. "And with all the extra space we're saving that used to be devoted to paper records, we can even add a new exam room now!"

- Most other physicians are excited about the new system, too. They are each happy about different benefits: the cost-savings they'll realize by reducing costs of paper charts and transcriptions, eliminating offsite storage costs, greater accuracy of prescription orders, and the ability to access records from home during evenings and weekends.

- Sally Sharp, FNP, agrees with Dr. Zeal about the benefits. "This new system is great!" she said. "It didn't take hardly any time at all to learn. Of course, learning new computer software has always come easy to me."

- Dr. Robert Rankle isn't nearly as enthusiastic. He's 72 years old and planning to retire next year. "I admit that I'm not technologically oriented," he said. "I can barely use computers, except for sending an occasional email to my grandkids." While continuing his protests, Dr. Rankle has been asking his secretary to transcribe notes and paste them into the EMR. In addition, he has decided not to use certain features of the EMR because "they're just too hard and it's not worth it to me to learn all the shortcuts and other stuff when I'd only use it for one year." Other physicians and the family nurse practitioners are upset about this; the entire group – including Dr. Rankle – decided to use the same core set of features when they discussed this new system a year ago.

- Two other physicians, Drs. Fine and Howard, often complain about the new system as well. They think the EMR is too difficult to use and that support services are so inadequate that minor issues often blow up into major ones.

- Darla DeTail is happy for the practice getting its new system, but she's a medical records technician and is fearful of losing her job. After all, it's a large practice and it seems that at least some of the medical record techs will be asked to go. Since Darla was the most recent to be hired, she suspects it will be her.

- Most billing staff members say that they've gone through the most difficult transition of anyone. Some say they're still getting used to Windows-based billing rather than DOS-based billing.

A nurse resents a
new physician's
attempts to change
procedures

Training Tool #89

Nursing wounds

TYPE: Case study

ESTIMATED TRAINING TIME: 30 minutes

THEMES: Organizational change, conflict management, negotiation

OBJECTIVE:

➡ to recognize that the timing and manner in which changes are made can have an effect on working relationships.

MATERIALS NEEDED: Copy of the two roles for each dyad

PROCEDURE:

Divide the group into dyads and ask one person to play the nurse, and the other to play the physician. Participants may change the character's first names if they would prefer to play a role in their own gender. Distribute a copy of the confidential instructions for each role so that each person in the dyad is playing a different role.

DEBRIEFING:

1 Was Dr. Miway justified in asking for certain procedures to be changed after first arriving? What are the pros and cons of making immediate changes to an existing practice?
2 Why was Ms. Haddinuff so upset about making changes in the charting system as Dr. Miway asked? Was it professional or appropriate for her to refuse to make the changes she was asked to make?
3 How would it be more likely for Dr. Miway to obtain Ms. Haddinuff's cooperation?
4 How could Ms. Haddinuff do a better job of conveying her concerns about the changes that the new doctor suggests?
5 What will both parties need to do to work together in the best interest of Genial Family Medicine?

CASE STUDY: NURSING WOUNDS

Iva Haddinuff, RN, has been with Genial Family Medicine for 10 years and has a great deal of influence over her coworkers. A new physician, Dr. Midas Miway, came to the practice three months ago. There are three other family physicians in the practice and Ms. Haddinuff has always gotten along with each of them very well.

Since Dr. Miway's arrival, he has asked to change several procedures, including major changes in the charting system. Ms. Haddinuff, who is very proud of the systems that she helped to develop, became extremely defensive when Dr. Miway suggested the changes. She told him why his changes wouldn't work and has steadfastly refused to take part in making them.

"He didn't even wait to learn our system first, or why we do things the way we do," Ms. Haddinuff told the office manager. The office manager said that it might be worth changing the systems – at least for a while – to see if Dr. Miway's methods work better for the practice.

Each time that Ms. Haddinuff has refused to comply, Dr. Miway raised his voice in disgust and then asks someone else to make the changes. Dr. Miway jokingly refers to Ms. Haddinuff throughout the office as "Attila the Hun" – a term that Ms. Haddinuff has heard around the office and absolutely doesn't like.

Training Tool #90

Introducing change

TYPE: Role play – five-persons: office manager, medical director, nurse, front office staff, and billing clerk

ESTIMATED TRAINING TIME: 90 minutes

THEMES: Organizational change, conflict management, negotiation

OBJECTIVES:
➡ to understand the importance of introducing change in an inclusive and methodical manner;
➡ to develop skills in resolving interpersonal problems that may arise when a controversial change is introduced.

MATERIALS NEEDED: A copy of the General Instructions for all participants, and a copy of the five character roles for each small group

PROCEDURE:
Ask participants to form into groups of five and distribute the General Instructions to everyone. Next, distribute the character roles so that each person in the small groups plays a different role. Note that they will have 40 minutes for the role-play discussion.

DEBRIEFING:
After the role plays, ask the following questions:
1 What was the outcome of your group's discussion in terms of (a) how the change will be handled; and (b) the effects on people's working relationships?
2 Did one or more "change managers" emerge in this exercise? If so, what roles did they play?
3 What were the positive and negative aspects of how the change was introduced (e.g. timing, methods, communication styles, etc.)?
4 What strategies were used to "sell" the change to group members? What other strategies might have worked better?
5 What was the level of resistance? How was it handled? Were strategies used that would help lead people through their typical emotional responses? What could have been done differently to reduce the level of resistance, either during or before this meeting?
6 Were efforts made to surface the underlying issues?
7 Were adjustments made to quell people's specific concerns about the change?

8 What other strategies could have been used to implement change more effectively?

9 Was there mention of personality differences between any of the characters? If so, how was this handled?

10 What lessons about organizational change will you be able to take away from this exercise?

Training Tool #90

ROLE PLAY: INTRODUCING CHANGE
GENERAL INSTRUCTIONS

Yellowfin Community Health Center (CHC) is a busy, productive practice, but relationships between leaders and some providers and staff members have been tense lately. Part of this may be due to the fact that one of the five physicians retired more than six months ago and still hasn't been replaced. Despite the medical director's recruitment efforts, only one candidate seemed viable so far, but she didn't want to live in Yellowfin. Meanwhile, the patient load has been exceptionally high.

The office manager has just called an all-hands meeting. Most staff members have heard a rumor that this will involve a new policy to keep the health center open one night a week – something that has not been done in the center's 15-year history. Leaders at Yellowfin CHC are enthusiastic about this change, but many providers and staff members are not. Some staff members have expressed concerns about not knowing the purpose of this meeting: Will they simply be told about the change? Will their input matter?

The players in your group represent the most vocal participants: the office manager, medical director, nurse, front office staff, and billing clerk. Before beginning the exercise, be sure to identify your role to other group members. You will have 40 minutes for this discussion. Consider the instructions about your role as a general guideline, but feel free to change course if you are influenced by the discussion – just as you would in real life.

ROLE PLAY: INTRODUCING CHANGE
CONFIDENTIAL INSTRUCTIONS

Office Manager

As the office manager at Yellowfin Community Health Center, you are about to announce to your staff that the center will now stay open until 9:00 pm every Thursday night. The medical director and the physicians are quite supportive of this change and the off-site administrator, who oversees four other clinics, is especially pleased. However, the rest of the staff doesn't know that this matter has already been decided. Now you need to sell the idea to them.

Along with the medical director and the physicians, you agree that it's essential to stay open at least one night a week. A recent study has shown a major increase in the number of two-parent working families in the area, and you have been concerned about numerous complaints from many of these families about accessibility to health care services. In addition to meeting community needs, you realize that staying open one night a week will result in a major increase in practice revenues. Because one of the physicians retired and hasn't yet been replaced for more than six months, the added revenues are more important than usual this year.

The majority of physicians were amenable to the idea of staying open one night a week anyway, but you thought it would only be fair to allow each physician one-half day off each week to make up for working on Thursday night. You do plan to pay time-and-a-half to administrative and front-office staff members who work evenings, but you don't plan to give them time off.

The medical director agreed with you that policy decisions such as this one did not require input from everyone in advance. Making today's announcement will be difficult; you've normally been a consensus builder in the past, but the medical director has often accused you of being too soft. Because several providers and staff members are upset about rumors regarding this plan, you secretly wonder if you might have been mistaken about making this decision without obtaining staff input first.

ROLE PLAY: INTRODUCING CHANGE
CONFIDENTIAL INSTRUCTIONS

Medical Director

As the medical director at Yellowfin Community Health Center, you're hoping that this change will go smoothly. You strongly support the idea of keeping the center open until 9:00 pm every Thursday night. In addition to meeting community needs, you believe that the extended hours will help to take pressure off the staff during daytime hours. Because one of your physician colleagues retired more than six months ago and hasn't yet been replaced, the schedule has been overloaded for months and there's no sign of it abating. You also like the idea that physicians will get a half day off during the week to make up for the extra night of work.

You can only see benefits from this change. Although you've heard that some administrative and front-line staff members aren't too happy about the idea because they wouldn't have time off – only overtime pay – this isn't of great concern to you. With many years of training and many long hours in practice over the years, you believe that you have paid your dues and that others should too. Besides, you see staff scheduling as the office manager's responsibility, not yours.

A few weeks ago, the office manager asked whether you thought the entire staff should be consulted on this matter in advance and you said no. In your opinion, organizations are not true democracies, and some policy decisions need to be made by leadership. Seeing the office manager take more control pleases you, as you've perceived that he/she hasn't had much spine. In several previous discussions, you've cautioned the office manager against being too soft.

ROLE PLAY: INTRODUCING CHANGE
CONFIDENTIAL INSTRUCTIONS

Nurse

As one of the nurse leaders at Yellowfin Community Health Center, you plan to speak up at today's all-staff meeting if the rumor about evening hours is true.

In addition to being upset about the extended hours, you are quite concerned with the process. You strongly believe that someone should have discussed this with you and other nurses in advance. (How can the center stay open during evening hours if nurses aren't present?) No matter what happens regarding the extended hours, you want assurances that nurses will be consulted in the future on matters that directly concern them.

You consider yourself a team player. You will work one night a week if you have to, but you don't like the idea and think it will just lead to staying open one more night and then another. You have two children, ages six months and two years. Your spouse doesn't like the idea that you won't be at home for even one night. When you talk to other nurses, most agree that time off and being able to achieve balance in one's life are far more important than extra pay.

You don't understand why patients can't just visit the hospital emergency room during evening hours. Another concern is why it is taking so long to recruit another physician to replace the one who retired. The medical director says that a candidate turned down an offer because she didn't like the community, but you don't buy it. You think it is due in large part to the medical director's style.

ROLE PLAY: INTRODUCING CHANGE
CONFIDENTIAL INSTRUCTIONS

Front-office Staff

You are a member of the front office staff of Yellowfin Community Health Center, and you're entering today's all-staff meeting with great trepidation. If management makes you work at night, you'll be furious. After all, when you took this job six years ago, it was with the understanding that you'd work days. In your mind, forcing you to work at night would be a violation of this verbal contract.

You have other things to do in the evenings and you don't want that time disturbed. For one thing, you serve as a volunteer for several community organizations and there are many people who depend on you to attend evening meetings. Most of your obligations fall on Thursday nights, so you would consider a request to work on that night to be the worst possible time.

You will be especially upset if you find out that the decision to keep the office open on Thursday night has already been made. Why didn't anybody ask for your input in advance? You need this job (it's your only source of income), but if the office manager and medical director insist that you work nights, you may just threaten to resign.

ROLE PLAY: INTRODUCING CHANGE
CONFIDENTIAL INSTRUCTIONS

Billing Clerk

As a billing clerk at Yellowfin Community Health Center, you are deeply concerned about the rumors that the center will stay open every Thursday evening until 9:00 pm. Several of your friends who work at night told you not to expect that you'll leave at 9:00 pm – that's probably when the last patient will be seen. Based on their experiences, they said to expect leaving at 10:00 pm or even later, after you and other staff members have straightened things up.

One reason this concerns you is that you don't like being out at night. About a year ago, a strange person approached you in the health center's parking lot. Thankfully, you were able to get to your car in time, but you've been a little nervous about that dimly lit parking lot ever since.

You're especially concerned about the hardship that this change will impose on your co-workers. Some are single parents and will have to find babysitters. Since the grapevine hasn't provided much information about the specifics, some of your co-workers are concerned about doing more work for the same amount of pay.

Despite these concerns, you consider yourself a reasonable person. If you're given convincing arguments that make sense to you and you feel that your needs (and those of your co-workers) are being addressed, you'll go along with the change. However, if you think that the arguments are flimsy or feel that you're being manipulated, you'll resist.

**Issues related to
the consolidation
of maternal and
pediatric services**

Training Tool #91

United we stand

TYPE: Role play and worksheet – two groups of employees

ESTIMATED TRAINING TIME: 90 minutes

THEME: Organizational change

OBJECTIVES:
➡ to learn skills in planning for an institutional change;
➡ to understand the need to plan for the change itself as well as the emotional and psychological aspects of change.

MATERIALS NEEDED: A copy of both the role play exercise and Change Worksheet for all participants

PROCEDURE:
In a brief lecture, tell participants about the importance of planning for change – not only strategizing about making the change itself, but also to plan for people's inevitable emotional and psychological reactions and helping them through their resistance.

Ask participants to form small groups and note that they will play the role of a team that will help the hospital to plan for both aspects of the change: structural and emotional.

Offer the worksheet as an aid for their planning of both aspects. Give the groups 45 minutes complete their plans.

DEBRIEFING:
1 Was the worksheet helpful in planning for both the structural and emotional/psychological aspects? If so, in what ways?
2 Why is it essential to plan for people's reactions as well as the change itself? Why do you think this aspect is often overlooked?
3 What did your group recommend in each planning component?
4 If this occurred in real life, how successful would your plan be in making the change and helping people through their resistance?

ROLE PLAY: UNITED WE STAND[7]

Your hospital administrator has asked you and other leaders of Holy Mackerel Hospital to serve on a committee to plan for the consolidation of maternal and pediatric services. The administrator believes that this is a wise move, as patient services through both areas will be more seamless, not to mention that it will result in major savings in overhead costs.

Your committee will need to plan for the change itself, but the most important part of today's meeting is to plan for people's emotional and psychological reactions to the change. As you plan for the change, realize that two services will be working together for the first time and several potential problems are likely to emerge:

- **Identity issues:** Those who currently practice in the maternal unit identify themselves with their adult patients, while those who practice in pediatrics identify with children. How can these two distinct "identities" be merged?

- **Loyalty issues:** Personnel are extremely loyal to the leaders of their respective services. What can be done to create loyalty to the new consolidated service? One of the heads of the two existing services will be named as the director of the consolidated service.

- **The "them-us syndrome":** Now that word has spread about the impending change, personnel from maternal and pediatric services are referring to one another as "us" and "them" more frequently. What can be done to create a new "us"?

- **Procedures:** Maternal and pediatric services each do things their own way and their procedures are very different. Should procedures be changed so that everyone in the consolidated unit is doing things the same way? Or should both services simply learn how the other does things and try to work out problems that may occur as a result of their differences?

---

7   Author's note: The idea for this case came from a scenario in a book by William Bridges, *Managing Transitions: Making the Most of Change*. Cambridge, MA: Perseus Books; 1991.

Change worksheet

CHANGE

Change:

(What change do you wish to make?)

Managing the Change Itself	Managing Emotional and Psychological Aspects
Likely Impacts:	
Systems and services:	Emotional reactions:
Process:	
(Kurt Lewin's change theory)	
Unfreezing: (Become motivated to change)	Letting go of the past:
Changing: (Change what needs to be changed)	Building stability:
Refreezing: (Making the change permanent)	Getting involved:
Strategies:	*Strategies:*
Vision for the change:	Denial, shock, grief:
Change champions:	Resistance to change:
Immediate needs:	Participation:

Managing the Change Itself	Managing Emotional and Psychological Aspects
Long-term needs:	Commitment:
Communication to implementers:	Reinforcement:
Decision making authority:	Recognition:

Communication:

Organizational:	Individual (performance level):
Group:	Individual (emotional, psychological):
Individual:	

Support:

Leadership support:	Leadership support:
Support from community partners:	Support from colleagues:
Other support:	Other support:

Communicating with emotional intelligence

Emotional intelligence: a vital skill for health care professionals

TYPE: Introductory discussion

ESTIMATED TRAINING TIME: 15 minutes

THEME: Emotional intelligence

OBJECTIVE:

➡ to create awareness about the importance of applying emotional intelligence skills in health care.

MATERIALS NEEDED: None

PROCEDURE:

After defining emotional intelligence and the four key competencies (self-awareness, self-management, social awareness, and relationship management), ask as many of the following questions as possible during the allotted time. (Allow more time if you plan a more extended lecture.)

1 Some say that, in many respects, emotional intelligence is more important than a person's IQ. Do you agree? Why or why not?

2 Do you believe that emotional intelligence should be included in the curricula of health professions training programs? Why or why not?

3 What are the applications of emotional intelligence in health care?

4 How does skill development in this area benefit health care professionals, staff members, patients, and others? Specifically, what are the effects in terms of decision making, communication, and relationships?

5 In general, which emotional intelligence competencies are strongest among members of your profession or discipline? Which are the weakest?

6 What are your own strengths and limitations? Which competencies do you want most to develop?

Training Tool #93

Self-management

TYPE: Introductory discussion

ESTIMATED TRAINING TIME: 15 minutes

THEMES: Emotional intelligence, conflict management, difficult colleagues, difficult conversations, communicating in crisis situations

OBJECTIVES:
➡ to identify options for the self-management of emotional reactions to situations in the workplace;
➡ to show that there are a variety of strategies for self-management of one's emotions.

MATERIALS NEEDED: Flip chart

PROCEDURE:
Ask the group the following questions and list their responses on the flip chart:
1 Think about difficult situations that you typically experience in your health care career as you deal with colleagues, patients, and others. What are some of the negative emotional reactions that you may feel when dealing with these situations? (Likely responses include anxious, tense, fearful, sad, and defensive.)
2 What might cause your emotional responses to escalate?
3 If your emotions are uncontrolled, what can happen? How might your communication with others be altered?
4 What do you normally do to manage your emotional responses? Which of your strategies work best?

DEBRIEFING:
Point out that while strategies for self-management are individualized, it may help to try some of the strategies suggested by other participants. Also explain that this discussion was intended to show that emotional responses are normal and controllable.

Identifying ways to
calm down others
who are angry or
upset

Giving emotional support

TYPE: Introductory discussion

ESTIMATED TRAINING TIME: 15 minutes

THEMES: Emotional intelligence, conflict management, difficult colleagues, difficult conversations, communicating in crisis situations

OBJECTIVE:
➥ to identify compassionate and helpful ways to respond to the emotional reactions of others (e.g. colleagues, patients).

MATERIALS NEEDED: Flip chart (optional)

PROCEDURE:
[Note: While Training Tool #93 addressed ways to manage a person's own emotions, this exercise is devoted to helping others with their emotional reactions.]

Provide an overview of the importance of the self-management component of emotional intelligence. Then point out that there are many ways to help others process their emotions and ask the group the following questions.

DEBRIEFING:
1 What strategies work best in these situations?
   ➥ A patient is crying uncontrollably.
   ➥ A patient is trembling, not because of temperature, but due to tension.
   ➥ An enraged colleague starts yelling at you.
   ➥ A colleague seems sad, preoccupied, and distressed.
2 What are some examples of things you should *not* say in response to someone's emotional reactions? (Possible responses: "You shouldn't feel that way!" "You have no need to cry." "I know exactly how you feel.") Explain the reasons for your responses.
3 What are your recommendations about touching? Hugging?
4 In what ways can you best show empathy for the other person?
5 What are your recommendations about giving emotional support to others when your time is limited?

Training Tool #95

Emotional recognition

TYPE: Introductory discussion

ESTIMATED TRAINING TIME: 30 minutes

THEME: Emotional intelligence

OBJECTIVES:

➡ to develop skills in deciphering the emotional state of others;

➡ to demonstrate the difficulty in identifying secondary and tertiary emotions in others.

MATERIALS NEEDED: Make one copy of the list of emotions on the next page and cut the page so there is one emotion on each strip. Put the strips in an envelope and mix them up.

PROCEDURE:

Ask for four or five volunteers to participate in a demonstration exercise. Then follow these steps:

➡ As the first volunteer comes to the front of the room, ask him/her to draw an emotion from the envelope, but without announcing it to the group.

➡ Instruct the volunteer to "act out" this emotion, noting that he/she may not use words and may only count (e.g. 1, 2, 3, 4, 5 . . .). Although volunteers may not use words, they may use their paralanguage (volume, rate, pitch, tone, pauses, and other vocal qualities), facial expressions, and body language to help others guess the emotion they are acting out.

➡ Tell participants to call out the emotion as soon as they identify it. The actor can stop only when someone accurately identifies the emotion or until the instructor stops the volunteer because no one has guessed the emotion they are trying to convey.

DEBRIEFING:

After each volunteer has acted out an emotion, ask the group:

1   Was the emotion easy or difficult to identify?

2   What did the actor do to convey the emotion with voice, facial expression, or body language?

3   What nonverbal cues were most helpful?

4   Which nonverbal cues were most confusing? If some were confusing, was the actor

giving mixed messages? (If some volunteers nervously smile as a reaction to being on stage, point out how mixed messages can increase the difficulty of interpretation.)

5   What does this exercise teach you about making untested assumptions about a person's emotional state?

At the conclusion of the exercise, point out that primary emotions (e.g. happiness, fear, and sadness) are normally the easiest to communicate and interpret accurately, while more complex (secondary and tertiary) emotions such as jealousy, love, and sympathy are more problematic because they often involve a combination of signals. Note that many complex emotions are more difficult to convey without directing the communication to another person.

Copy this page and cut on the lines (also down the middle) so that there is one emotion on each strip. Place the strips in an envelope and mix them up.

Happy	Sad
Fear	Anxiety
Anxiety	Disgust
Anger	Apprehensive
Love	Hate
Guilt	Jealous
Sympathy	Alienated
Embarrassed	Ashamed
Dread	Surprised
Depressed	Resentful

Three case studies
to apply emotional
intelligence
competencies

Case studies in emotional intelligence

TYPE: Case studies

ESTIMATED TRAINING TIME: 45 minutes each

THEME: Emotional intelligence

OBJECTIVE:

➡ to apply the four competencies in emotional intelligence to a situation involving health care professionals.

MATERIALS NEEDED: A copy of the selected case study for all participants

PROCEDURE:

Ask participants to form small groups and read the selected case study. Note that they will be asked to determine what they will do or say to ensure that they would handle the situation in an emotionally intelligent way by incorporating the four emotional intelligence competencies into their handling of the case. Tell the small groups to allow 30 minutes for their discussion, and that the remaining time will be devoted to an all-group discussion.

Your choices of case studies are as follows:

➡ **Family feud** – Your family is upset that you are spending too much time away from them.

➡ **Perceived persecution** – A defensive employee who receives a poor performance appraisal believes that the evaluation was unfair.

➡ **Out of sync** – A resident's catastrophic personal problems have become manifested in some disturbing behaviors.

Point out that the group should answer the list of questions that appear after the case and be prepared to discuss them with the group as a whole.

DEBRIEFING:

Identify similarities and dissimilarities among the responses from each group and close the session with a reiteration of key learning points.

CASE STUDY: FAMILY FEUD

Your spouse refers to you as a workaholic, and you admit it. You love your work! You get up earlier than most people, go to work before the sun rises (you're the one who opens the doors to the practice) and work on your computer until patients begin to arrive. After a full day of practice, you often attend meetings of the several Boards of Directors you serve on (including those that deal with breast cancer research and multiple sclerosis). You also make routine visits to a nearby long-term care facility.

"Enough is enough," your spouse now says, angrily. "You can't seem to say 'no' to anyone except for your family. Our daughter refers to you as an absentee parent! No wonder she is having so many problems in school."

You do not wish to cut back on what you do, and enjoy your demanding career. You feel that your daughter gets plenty of your attention on weekends and you don't understand what your spouse is so upset about. What's the big deal about having meals with you?

DISCUSSION QUESTIONS

Self-awareness

- What would you need to be introspective about in order to deal with this situation?
- What emotions would you be likely to experience?
- What are your gut feelings about this situation?
- What would be the impact on others of having a negative emotional response?

Self-management

- What would you do to control your own emotions and impulses while discussing this matter with your spouse?
- What would you do if your spouse reacted in an unexpected manner, e.g. with warnings, threats or ultimatums?

Social-awareness

- Other than your spouse and child, what other persons are likely to be affected by the results of your discussion?
- What, if anything, is the relationship between the time you spend on your professional career and your daughter's problems in school?
- What emotions are your spouse and daughter likely to be experiencing as a result of this dilemma?
- Could there be underlying issues involving your spouse's or daughter's

concerns about your time away from the family? If so, what might some of those be?

Relationship management

▶ What will your goal be? Will it be to persuade your family to accept your hectic schedule? Will you make minor accommodations? Major ones? Include your family in some of your professional events?

▶ How will you handle the conversation with your spouse about this matter? How important are listening skills?

▶ In addition to resolving the issue (i.e. the use of your time), what will you do or say to improve your relationship with your spouse? How will you acknowledge your spouse's strong feelings about this matter?

▶ What will you say or do differently with your daughter? What will you do to explore your daughter's feelings?

CASE STUDY: PERCEIVED PERSECUTION

You are about to have a follow-up discussion with one of your employees, Lisa Marie Peasley. It was only last week that you gave her a very poor performance appraisal for her work in the practice's administrative office. You cited the problems as: too much horsing around and chit-chatting with other employees; not completing assignments on time; and making too many mistakes. During the performance appraisal, you decided to put Lisa Marie on probation.

Ever since the appraisal, Lisa Marie has been very angry and hasn't been shy about her feelings to everyone else in the office. She believes you were extremely unfair because you focused on everything she does wrong rather than all the good work she has done for the practice. She also says you're ungrateful; after all, it was her father who started the practice many years ago (he has since passed away, although some people still feel his presence), and there's even a portrait of him in the reception area.

At today's follow-up meeting, you would like for Lisa Marie to "own" the problems she has created and to improve her performance. You do NOT want to let her go as you are extremely short-staffed right now – not to mention that you don't want to be known as the person who fired Dr. Peasley's daughter.

DISCUSSION QUESTIONS

Self-awareness
▶ What would you need to be introspective about in order to deal with this situation?
▶ What emotions would you be likely to experience?
▶ What are your gut feelings about this situation?
▶ What would be the impact on Lisa Marie and others if you should have a negative emotional response?

Self-management
▶ What would you do to control your own emotions and impulses while discussing this matter with Lisa Marie, especially given her anger?
▶ What would you do if Lisa Marie reacted by threatening to resign – or if she handed you her resignation letter?

Social-awareness
▶ Other than Lisa Marie, who else is being affected by this situation both within and outside of the office?
▶ What is the likely effect of Lisa Marie's anger on her coworkers?

- What emotions is it likely that Lisa Marie has been experiencing before and after the performance evaluation?
- Could there be underlying issues? If so, what might some of those be?
- Does it matter that Lisa Marie's father helped to create the practice and is well-regarded throughout the community? Please explain.

Relationship management
- What will your goals be in your conversation with Lisa Marie other than to encourage her to improve her performance?
- What will you do or say to deal with Lisa Marie's emotions?
- What will you do or say to influence her to improve her performance?
- Is it important to help Lisa Marie save face? If so, why? How? With whom?

CASE STUDY: OUT OF SYNC

As the Director of Behavioral Science at your Family Medicine Residency Program, you are quite concerned with the behavior of one of your residents, Rose Blackwater, MD. You know this has been a rough time for Rose; her fiancé, Jack Lawson, was lost at sea during a recent cruise they took together. She came back alone – at first inconsolable, and later in a state of shock and disbelief. In addition to losing the love of her life, Rose is tremendously upset that she doesn't know exactly what happened. Did Jack fall overboard? Did he throw himself out to sea? Did someone push him? Rose was questioned by the authorities for what seemed like weeks, but Jack's death was determined to be accidental. She doesn't know what she's reacting to more: losing Jack, not knowing what happened to him, or seeming to be accused of being involved in his disappearance. She feels better now that she is working once again.

It's now a little more than a month after the catastrophic incident, and Rose is often seen either staring blankly at people or gazing out of the window for long periods of time. Faculty members are getting annoyed that they have to repeat things to Rose several times; why doesn't she listen to them the first time? Other residents are noticing that Rose tends to isolate herself; she won't even have lunch with them and doesn't seem to engage in small talk. She is quite sullen, even though you know she is taking an antidepressant. The residency director has recently talked with you about Rose's behavior, but noted that there have not been major problems with her productivity or performance. You have decided to talk with her today.

DISCUSSION QUESTIONS

Self-awareness

▶ What would you need to be introspective about in order to deal with this situation?

▶ What emotions would you be likely to experience?

▶ What are your gut feelings about this situation?

▶ As long as Rose is keeping up with her work and doing reasonably well, what would be your reasons for discussing Rose's behavior with her?

Self-management

▶ How do you plan to begin the discussion with Rose?

▶ What would you believe is most important to say to Rose during this difficult time? What types of things should you NOT say?

▶ What would you do if Rose behaves in an erratic or unexpected manner?

▶ How would you demonstrate empathy and concern for her wellbeing?

Social-awareness

▶ Which parties in the residency are likely to be affected by Rose's behavior? What other parties are likely to be affected?

▶ What will you look for in Rose during this conversation? The extent of her depression? Whether she would do something to act out her grief? What else?

▶ What emotions do you think that Rose might experience during your conversation?

▶ Does it matter which issue is bothering Rose more – the loss of Jack, not knowing what happened to him, or being interrogated? Explain your response.

Relationship management

▶ What will your goals be for your conversation with Rose? To let her know you are there for her? To convince her to change behaviors?

▶ What will you tell the residency director about your conversation with Rose? If Rose asks to speak in confidence, what would you say then?

▶ What would you say, if anything, to faculty members and residents about what Rose is going through?

▶ Would you recommend that Rose take more time off, even though she has been away for more than a month?

Applying emotional intelligence competencies to two situations

Training Tools #99–100

Role plays – emotional intelligence

TYPE: Role play

ESTIMATED TRAINING TIME: 60 minutes

THEME: Emotional intelligence

OBJECTIVE:

- to practice using skills in emotional intelligence through role play exercises.

MATERIALS NEEDED: A copy of the two roles (A and B) for each dyad

PROCEDURE:

Ask the group to form dyads and distribute the instructions so that one is given the A sheet and the other receives the B sheet. They will each play the roles on this sheet for both exercises. Tell the group that they will have 30 minutes to act out the two cases; the remaining time will be devoted to an all-group discussion. The two role plays that will be conducted during the time frame are:

- **Up in smoke** – A patient with smoke on her breath denies what she's done.
- **Bad chemistry** – A nurse questions a physician assistant about a possible medication error.

DEBRIEFING:

For each case, ask the group to address the following questions:

1. In addition to substantive issues, what were the emotional issues for each player?
2. Did these layers get confused? If so, how?
3. What verbal and nonverbal cues informed you about the other party's emotions? Were your assessments accurate?
4. How did the emotional undercurrents complicate the situation?
5. Did both parties openly discuss the emotional component of their conversation or did this aspect remain tacit?
6. What emotional intelligence competencies would be most helpful for the clinician in each case?

ROLE PLAYS: EMOTIONAL INTELLIGENCE
PLAYER A

#99: "Up in Smoke"

You are a family physician who is now meeting with a 51-year-old patient you've seen for more than 10 years, Mrs. Hilda Huffinpuff. Long before diagnosing her coronary artery disease, you advised Mrs. Huffinpuff to stop smoking and provided her with several smoking cessation tools and hours of personal counseling. For the last four months, she has maintained that she quit smoking, but on today's visit you smell tobacco and mouthwash on her breath. Nothing presses your hot buttons more than people who lie to your face.

#100: "Bad Chemistry"

You are Nellie Neely, RN, a nurse who began working at the Greenplace Community Health Center five years ago, just as the center opened. Although you generally like your job, you are quite distressed about your poor working relationship with the physician assistant who has been there for a year now. You don't remember anyone ever treating you with such disdain! You know that the physician assistant treats you differently than other nurses, frequently accusing you of looking for mistakes when you've asked simple questions for clarification. While you think that the physician assistant is too quick to jump on you for the slightest thing, you've asked to meet today to discuss a possible medication error that the physician assistant seems to have made. You could be wrong, but you think that the dosage is too high. Although you're afraid of being accused of second-guessing the physician assistant again, you'd feel remiss in your responsibilities if you didn't ask.

ROLE PLAYS: EMOTIONAL INTELLIGENCE
PLAYER B

#99: "Up in Smoke"

You are Mrs. Hilda Huffinpuff, aged 51 and a heavy smoker. Today, you are seeing your family physician of 10 years on a follow-up visit related to your coronary artery disease. After years of pleading, your doctor convinced you to quit smoking, which you almost did four months ago. Although you are still smoking, you don't want to tell the doctor about it. Not only would you lose face, you are afraid the doctor won't like or respect you anymore. You smoked quite a bit this morning – you were paying bills, after all – but covered up traces with mouthwash and breath mints. If the doctor asks about smoking, you'll deny it as usual. If forced to admit your habit, you have plenty of excuses in store.

#100: "Bad Chemistry"

You are a physician assistant and have been at the Greenplace Community Health Center for one year. You can't quite put your finger on all the reasons, but you don't care for one of the nurses, Nellie Neely, RN, who joined the practice five years ago, when it started. You frequently feel that Nellie is looking over your shoulder, just waiting until you make a mistake so that she can report you to administration. When you've mentioned your suspicions about her motives in the past, she has denied trying to second-guess your judgment, and has said that she's simply asking questions for clarification, just as any good nurse would do. Nellie has just asked to speak to you privately, and you are gritting your teeth just thinking of another confrontation. You realize that you treat her differently than other nurses, but there's something about Nellie that rubs you the wrong way. You hope she isn't going to point out a mistake you made on a prescription by writing down the wrong dosage. Another nurse caught the mistake and you thanked her for pointing it out, but you don't want to address this matter with Nellie.

Tips for trainers

➡ **Select a private room for training activities.** Test any audio-visual equipment before the program. Keep an extra bulb on hand for overhead projectors. Ask participants to use "vibrating" beepers in order to avoid distractions.

➡ **Do your homework.** If you are training 10 health care professionals in a one-hour session, realize that you're utilizing 10 total hours of people's time – and that's an investment. Make their time count by developing a well-structured agenda and doing the necessary research in advance.

➡ **Vary your activities.** The experiential approach ("learning-by-doing") is an excellent way to provide training in communication-related strategies. Incorporate several training methods into your program by using a combination of activities, such as didactic presentations, self-tests, films, role-playing exercises, case studies, group discussions, problem-solving sessions, and audio-visual presentations.

➡ **Encourage participants to "stretch."** When role-playing, some participants may balk at playing the roles of persons in other specialties, professions, or disciplines. If this occurs, you can either modify the exercises to suit the participants, or ask participants to put themselves in their respective character's shoes. Explain that this will help them see the conflict from another party's perspective.

➡ **Be a good teacher.** When presenting a didactic lecture, make your points come alive by using metaphors and relevant examples. Explain new terminology. Use visual aids as appropriate. Lace your talk with humor to keep your audience awake and interested.

➡ **Be a good facilitator.** One of the best ways to ensure a good learning experience is to help participants process the lessons from each exercise through well-facilitated group discussions. Vary the pace of the program, ask "answerable" questions, summarize points, and keep things moving. Be sure to allow for a sufficient amount of discussion time before rushing to the next activity.

➡ **Evaluate the training session.** At the conclusion of the program, ask participants to complete an evaluation form so that you can improve future training programs. Keep the form brief, with questions such as: Was this program helpful to you? Why or why not? What did you find most beneficial . . . and the least? What suggestions do you have for future training topics? Any other comments or suggestions?

The art of giving critiques

When doing role-play exercises, participants will learn through their participation as well as through critiques by the instructor and other trainees. To ensure that participants will be receptive to these critiques, it's important to avoid embarrassing, hurting, or offending those who need to improve their skills in certain areas. Anyone who is asked to critique others should consider these suggestions.

➡ **Remember: critiques are to reinforce the positives too!**

It's not uncommon for people to think of critiques as telling others what they didn't do as well as they should or what they need to improve upon. That's part of it, but not all. Critiques are also for the purpose of explaining what others do well, as that will encouraged them to continue using those practices in the future. So don't forget to reinforce the strengths that you see in others!

➡ **Make observations, not conclusions**

To show the difference between these two concepts, an observation would be "You're late" while a conclusion would be "You're irresponsible!" Applying this to critiques, be sure that you explain what you saw the other party do or what you heard them say that needs to be tweaked or improved. Avoid making blanket statements that appear to be a conclusion about the other person.

➡ **Criticize the act, not the person**

Parents today learn that they shouldn't say, "Billy, you're a bad boy," because Billy is not a bad person – he just did something wrong. Modern day parents are advised to say instead, "Billy, you're a great kid and I love you – but your behavior right now is unacceptable!" We need to do the same thing when giving effective critiques: separate the people from the problem. If a trainee needs to improve a skill, mention what needs to be improved, but don't diminish the person in the process.

➡ **Keep comments professional, not emotional**

Critique sessions aren't the time to get back at a colleague for things they've done or said in the past. The focus needs to be on the exercise under discussion. Keep the discussion professional and make it a point to avoid confusing the discussion with old emotional baggage.

➡ **Concentrate on improving skills, not placing blame**

The learning curve will vary for all of those who engage in training exercises as they try to learn new skills and discard old habits that don't work in their favor. Don't blame them for their missteps; remember that this is a learning atmosphere and that people learn as much from their mistakes as they do their successes!

Quotations on training topics

[Note: These topics are listed in the same order that the exercises appear throughout the book.]

CONFLICT MANAGEMENT

"The most intense conflicts, if overcome, leave behind a sense of security and calm that is not easily disturbed. It is just these intense conflicts and their conflagration which are needed to produce valuable and lasting results." – Carl Jung

"Whenever you're in conflict with someone, there is one factor that can make the difference between damaging your relationship and deepening it. That factor is attitude." – Timothy Bentley

"You can't shake hands with a clenched fist." – Indira Gandhi

"How many a dispute could have been deflated into a single paragraph if the disputants had dared to define their terms?" – Aristotle

"People who fight with fire usually end up with ashes." – Abigail Van Buren

"Man must evolve for all human conflict a method which rejects revenge, aggression, and retaliation." – Martin Luther King, Jr.

"Conflict can be seen as a gift of energy, in which neither side loses and a new dance is created." – Thomas Crum

"When elephants fight, it is the grass who suffers." – African proverb

NEGOTIATING STRATEGIES – BARGAINING

"You got to be very careful if you don't know where you're going, because you might not get there." – Yogi Berra

"A good deal is a state of mind." – Lee Iococca

"My father said: you must never try to make all the money that's in a deal. Let the other fellow make some money too, because if you have a reputation for always making all the money, you won't have many deals." – J Paul Getty

"Negotiating in the classic diplomatic sense assumes parties are more anxious to agree than disagree." – Dean Acheson

DEALING WITH DIFFICULT COLLEAGUES

"... there is a good side and a bad side to most people, and in accordance with your own character and disposition you will bring out one of them and the other will remain a sealed book to you." – Mark Twain

"I don't like that man very much ... I'm going to have to get to know him better." – Abraham Lincoln, [attributed]

"Fix the problem, not the blame." – Japanese proverb

"I argue very well. Ask any of my remaining friends. I can win an argument on any topic, against any opponent. People know this, and steer clear of me at parties. Often, as a sign of their great respect, they don't even invite me." – Dave Barry

"Always forgive your enemies – nothing annoys them so much." – Oscar Wilde

"I told my psychiatrist that everyone hates me. He said I was being ridiculous – everyone hasn't met me yet." – Rodney Dangerfield

DIFFICULT CONVERSATIONS

"When you are kind to someone in trouble, you hope they'll remember and be kind to someone else. And it'll become like wildfire." – Whoopi Goldberg

"So long as you can sweeten another's pain, life is not in vain." – Helen Keller

"When you listen with empathy to another person, you give that person psychological air." – Stephen R Covey

COMMUNICATING IN CRISIS SITUATIONS

"Next week there can't be any crisis. My schedule is already full." – Henry Kissinger

"Every little thing counts in a crisis." – Jawaharlal Nehru

"In a crisis, don't hide behind anything or anybody. They're going to find you anyway." – Bear Bryant

"The Chinese use two brush strokes to write the word 'crisis.' One brush stroke stands for danger; the other for opportunity. In a crisis, be aware of the danger, but recognize the opportunity." – John F Kennedy

"It's not whether you get knocked down. It's whether you get up again." – Vince Lombardi

"The ultimate measure of a man is not where he stands in moments of comfort and convenience, but where he stands at times of challenge and controversy." – Martin Luther King

"To be mature means to face, and not evade, every fresh crisis that comes." – Fritz Kunkel

DEALING WITH ORGANIZATIONAL CHANGE

"Change is not merely necessary to life, it is life." – Alvin Toffler

"You must be the change you wish to see in the world." –Mahatma Gandhi

"Nothing endures but change." – Heraclitus

"There is a certain relief in change, even though it be from bad to worse; as I have found in traveling in a stagecoach, that it is often a comfort to shift one's position and be bruised in a new place." – Washington Irving, *Tales of a Traveler*

"There's only one person who likes change: a baby getting a new diaper." – Unknown

COMMUNICATING WITH EMOTIONAL INTELLIGENCE

"Emotional intelligence, more than any other factor, more than I.Q. or expertise, accounts for 85% to 90% of success at work . . . I.Q. is a threshold competence. You need it, but it doesn't make you a star. Emotional intelligence can." – Warren Bennis

"Let's not forget that the little emotions are the great captains of our lives and we obey them without realizing it." – Vincent Van Gogh

"People who fly into a rage always make a bad landing." – Will Rogers

"What really matters for success, character, happiness, and life long achievements is a definite set of emotional skills – your EQ – not just purely cognitive abilities that are measured by conventional IQ tests." – Daniel Goleman

"Comparing the three domains, I found that for jobs of all kinds, emotional competencies were twice as prevalent among distinguishing competencies as were technical skills and purely cognitive abilities combined. In general, the higher a position in an organization, the more EI mattered: for individuals in leadership positions, 85% of their competencies were in the EI domain." – Daniel Goleman

Matrix 1: Exercises by training subject

Title	Page	Conflict management	Negotiating strategies
Conflict management			
1 Five professional goals	3	X	X
2 Dissecting a common conflict	5	X	
3 What are your hot buttons?	6	X	X
4 First reactions	7	X	X
5 Healthy vs unhealthy conflict	8	X	
6 Word association and conflict	10	X	
7 Turf wars	12	X	X
8 Generational conflict	14	X	
9 Not my job	17	X	X
10 Moonlight in your eyes	19	X	X
11 A disheartening situation	21	X	X
12 Letting bygones be bygones	23	X	
13 The Doctor-in-the-Brochure	26	X	X
14 What is fair?	30	X	X
15 The joker is wild	31	X	
16 Building bonds	32	X	
17 Medicine woman	33	X	
18 Mars and Venus	34	X	

Difficult colleagues	Difficult conversations	Crises	Organizational change	Emotional intelligence
X	X	X	X	X
X	X	X	X	X
X				
X				
X				
			X	
X				X
X				
X				
	X			
X				

Title	Page	Conflict management	Negotiating strategies
19 Gender bias	35	X	
20 A dose of reality	36	X	X
21 It's your call	43	X	X
22 The paper chase	46	X	X
23 Clinically speaking	49	X	
24 Question of priorities	52	X	X
25 Preferential treatment	55	X	
26 A toxic situation	58	X	X
27 The Divisions' dilemma	61	X	X
28 Expansion plans	64	X	X
29 FamCare: difference in perspectives	67	X	X
30 Changing roles	69	X	X
31 The recalcitrant resident	71	X	X
32 Shifting resources in a state health agency	76	X	X
33 Special delivery	79	X	X
34 Working hand-in-hand	82	X	X
Negotiating-bargaining			
35 Future uses of negotiation	87		X
36 Empty chair	88		X
37 Negotiation self-test	89		X

Difficult colleagues	Difficult conversations	Crises	Organizational change	Emotional intelligence
X				
X				
X				
X				
X				
X				

Difficult colleagues	Difficult conversations	Crises	Organizational change	Emotional intelligence
X				
X				
X				
X				
X				X
X				X

Title	Page	Conflict management	Negotiating strategies
57 Better late than never	165	X	
58 The Mount Vesuvius effect	167	X	X
59 Oyl and Water	170	X	
60 Jack the Ripper	172	X	
61 Questionable source	174		
62 The Wright stuff	176	X	
Difficult conversations			
63 Challenging conversations	181		
64 A hairy problem	183		
65 Added stress	184		
66 Motor mouth	185		
67 Lay off	186		
68 Adding insult to injury	187		
69 Dress code	188		
70 Shocking news	189		
71 Consoling thoughts	193		
72 A malignant situation	196		
73 It's hard to say	199		
74 Getting ahead	202		
75 The nose knows	205		
76 Cloud of suspicion	208		

Difficult colleagues	Difficult conversations	Crises	Organizational change	Emotional intelligence
X				
X				X
X				
X				X
X	X			
X				
	X			
	X			
	X			
	X			
	X			
	X			
	X			
	X			X
	X			
	X			
	X			
	X			
	X			
	X			

Difficult colleagues	Difficult conversations	Crises	Organizational change	Emotional intelligence
		X		
		X		
		X		
		X		
		X		
		X		
		X		
		X		
			X	
			X	
			X	
			X	
			X	
			X	
			X	
				X
X	X	X	X	X

Difficult colleagues	Difficult conversations	Crises	Organizational change	Emotional intelligence
X	X	X	X	X
				X
	X			X
X	X			X
	X			X
	X			X
X				X

Matrix 2: Exercises by profession

Nurse	Physician assistant	Administrator	Public health	Other
				X
X				
		X		
X				
X	X	X		
X				X
				X
X				

Nurse	Physician assistant	Administrator	Public health	Other
X				
		X		
		X		
		X		X
			X	X
			X	
		X		
			X	
			X	
			X	

Nurse	Physician assistant	Administrator	Public health	Other
				X
		X		
		X		
				X
		X		
		X		
			X	
			X	
X				X
				X
X				

Nurse	Physician assistant	Administrator	Public health	Other
X				
	X			

Nurse	Physician assistant	Administrator	Public health	Other
X	X		X	
X				
		X		X
X				
		X		X

Nurse	Physician assistant	Administrator	Public health	Other
X				
		X		X
		X		X
X				
X		X		

Nurse	Physician assistant	Administrator	Public health	Other
		X		X
				X
X	X			

Matrix 3: Exercises by time allotment

Note: A number in parentheses tells how many exercises are included in that training time.

Title	Page	15 minutes	30 minutes	45 minutes	60 minutes	90 minutes
Conflict management						
1 Five professional goals	3	X				
2 Dissecting a common conflict	5	X				
3 What are your hot buttons?	6	X				
4 First reactions	7	X				
5 Healthy vs unhealthy conflict	8	X				
6 Word association and conflict	10	X				
7 Turf wars	12		X			
8 Generational conflict	14		X			
9 Not my job	17		X			
10 Moonlight in your eyes	19		X			
11 A disheartening situation	21		X			

Title	Page	15 minutes	30 minutes	45 minutes	60 minutes	90 minutes
12 Letting bygones be bygones	23		X			
13 The Doctor-in-the-Brochure	26				X	
14 What is fair?	30		X(2)			
15 The joker is wild	31		X(2)			
16 Building bonds	32		X(2)			
17 Medicine woman	33		X(2)			
18 Mars and Venus	34		X(2)			
19 Gender bias	35		X(2)			
20 A dose of reality	36					X
21 It's your call	43		X			
22 The paper chase	46		X			
23 Clinically speaking	49		X			
24 A question of priorities	52		X			
25 Preferential treatment	55		X			
26 A toxic situation	58			X		
27 The Divisions' dilemma	61				X	
28 Expansion plans	64				X	

Title	Page	15 minutes	30 minutes	45 minutes	60 minutes	90 minutes
29 FamCare: difference in perspectives	67		X			
30 Changing roles	69		X			
31 The recalcitrant resident	71				X	
32 Shifting resources in a state health agency	76		X			
33 Special delivery	79				X	
34 Working hand-in-hand	82			X		

Negotiating-bargaining

Title	Page	15 minutes	30 minutes	45 minutes	60 minutes	90 minutes
35 Future uses of negotiation	87	X				
36 Empty chair	88	X				
37 Negotiation self-test	89		X			
38 Framing issues	95			X		
39 Family practice/ managed care contract dilemma	98		X			
40 Let's renegotiate	101		X			
41 My way or the highway	103		X			
42 The squabbling doctors	106		X			

Title	Page	15 minutes	30 minutes	45 minutes	60 minutes	90 minutes
43 A new lease on life	110		X			
44 A salary negotiation	113				X	
45 The contract deadline	118				X	
46 An interagency agreement	122					X
47 Hot topic	128					X
48 Picture perfect	137		X			
49 Lab work	140			X		
50 The medical home	144				X	
51 Negotiation at Frugality Hospital	146				X	
52 The hidden agenda	149		X			
Difficult colleagues						
53 Reflecting on a difficult behavior	155		X			
54 Dealing with difficult behaviors	157		X			
55 Sticks and stones	159		X			
56 The e-tantrum	161	X				

Title	Page	15 minutes	30 minutes	45 minutes	60 minutes	90 minutes
57 Better late than never	165		X			
58 The Mount Vesuvius effect	167		X			
59 Oyl and Water	170		X			
60 Jack the Ripper	172		X			
61 Questionable source	174		X			
62 The Wright stuff	176		X			

Difficult conversations

Title	Page	15 minutes	30 minutes	45 minutes	60 minutes	90 minutes
63 Challenging conversations	181	X				
64 A hairy problem	183		X(2)			
65 Added stress	184		X(2)			
66 Motor mouth	185		X(2)			
67 Lay off	186		X(2)			
68 Adding insult to injury	187		X(2)			
69 Dress code	188		X(2)			
70 Shocking news	189		X			
71 Consoling thoughts	193					X(3)
72 A malignant situation	196					X(3)
73 It's hard to say	199					X(3)

Title	Page	15 minutes	30 minutes	45 minutes	60 minutes	90 minutes
74 Getting ahead	202					X(3)
75 The nose knows	205					X(3)
76 Cloud of suspicion	208					X(3)
Communicating in crisis situations						
77 The potential for crises	213	X				
78 From bad to worse	214	X				
79 Signal detection	215		X			
80 Heard it through the grapevine	218				X(2)	
81 Inevitable outcome	219				X(2)	
82 A scary world	221				X(2)	
83 Oh, rats!	223				X(2)	
84 Crisis response	225				X	
Organizational change						
85 My personal experience with change	229	X				
86 Changes in an interdependent system	231		X			
87 An association in turmoil	232		X			

Title	Page	15 minutes	30 minutes	45 minutes	60 minutes	90 minutes
88 When software is hard	234		X			
89 Nursing wounds	236		X			
90 Introducing change	238					X
91 United we stand	246					X
Emotional intelligence						
92 Emotional intelligence in health care	253	X				
93 Self-management	254	X				
94 Giving emotional support	255	X				
95 Emotional recognition	256		X			
96 Family feud	260			X		
97 Perceived persecution	262			X		
98 Out of sync	264			X		
99 Up in smoke	267				X(2)	
100 Bad chemistry	267				X(2)	

Suggested reading

CONFLICT MANAGEMENT (Also see books on negotiation and difficult colleagues)

Aries E. *Men and Women in Interaction: reconsidering the differences.* New York: Oxford University Press; 1996.

Fisher R, Brown S. *Getting Together: building a relationship that gets to yes.* Boston: Houghton Mifflin Company; 1988.

Gerzon M. *Leading Through Conflict: how successful leaders transform differences into opportunities.* Boston: Harvard Business School Press; 2006.

Haden Elgin S. *Genderspeak: men, women, and gentle art of self-defense.* New York: John Wiley & Sons; 1993.

Kolb DM, Partunek JM, editors. *Hidden Conflict in Organizations: uncovering behind-the-scenes disputes.* Newbury Park: Sage Publications; 1992.

Marcus LJ, Dorn B, Kritek, PB, *et al. Renegotiating Health Care: resolving conflict to build collaboration.* San Francisco: Jossey-Bass Publishers; 1995.

Susskind L, Cruikshank J. *Breaking the Impasse: consensual approaches to resolving public disputes.* New York: Basic Books, Inc.; 1987.

NEGOTIATING STRATEGIES – BARGAINING

Bazerman MH, Neale MA. *Negotiating Rationally.* New York: The Free Press; 1992.

Chambers R, editor. *Making an Effective Bid: a practical guide for research, teaching, and consultancy.* Abingdon, UK: Radcliffe Publishing; 2007.

Cohen S. *Negotiating Skills for Managers.* New York: McGraw Hill; 2002.

Fisher R, Ury W. *Getting to Yes: negotiating agreement without giving in.* Harrisonburg, VA: RR Donnelley & Sons Company; 1985.

Kolb D, Williams J. *The Shadow Negotiation: how women can master the hidden agendas that determine bargaining success.* New York: Simon & Schuster; 2000.

Kolb D, Williams J. *Everyday Negotiation: navigating the hidden agendas in bargaining.* San Francisco: Jossey-Bass; 2003.

Lax DA, Sebenius JK. *3D Negotiation: powerful tools to change the game in your most important deals.* Boston, MA: Harvard Business School Press; 2006.

Lewicki RJ, Hiam A, Olander KW. *Think Before You Speak: a complete guide to strategic negotiation.* New York: John Wiley & Sons; 1996.

Malhotra D, Bazerman M. *Negotiation Genius: how to overcome obstacles and achieve brilliant results at the bargaining table and beyond.* New York: Bantam Books; 2007.

Shell R. *Bargaining for Advantage: negotiation strategies for reasonable people.* New York: Penguin Books; 1999.

Thompson L. *The Mind and Heart of the Negotiator.* 4th ed. Upper Saddle River, NJ: Prentice Hall; 2001.

Ury W. *Getting Past No: negotiating with difficult people.* New York: Bantam Books; 1991.

Watkins M. *Shaping the Game: the new leader's guide to effective negotiating.* Boston: Harvard Business School Press; 2006.

DEALING WITH DIFFICULT COLLEAGUES

Gill L. *How to Work With Just About Anyone: a 3-step solution for getting difficult people to change.* New York: Simon and Schuster; 1999.

Horn S. *Tongue Fu!: how to deflect, disarm, and defuse any verbal conflict.* New York: St. Martin's Press; 1996.

Horn S. *Take the Bully by the Horns: stop unethical, uncooperative, or unpleasant people from running and ruining your life.* New York: St. Martin's Press; 2002.

Lloyd K. *Jerks at Work: how to deal with people problems and problem people.* Franklin Lakes, NJ: Career Press; 1999.

Pachter B. *The Power of Positive Confrontation: the skills you need to know to handle conflicts at work, home, and in life.* New York: Marlowe and Company; 2000.

Thistlethwaite J, Spencer J. *Professionalism in Medicine.* Abingdon, UK: Radcliffe Publishing; 2008.

Ury W. *Getting Past No: negotiating with difficult people.* New York: Bantam Books; 1993.

DIFFICULT CONVERSATIONS

Donovan C, Suckling H, Walker Z, *et al. Difficult Consultations with Adolescents.* Abingdon, UK: Radcliffe Publishing; 2004.

Faulkner A. *When the News is Bad: a guide for health professionals.* Cheltenham, UK: Stanley Thornes Publishers, Ltd.; 1998.

Gilbert M. *Communication Miracles at Work: effective tools and tips for getting the most from your work relationships.* Berkeley, CA: Conari Press; 2002.

Guilmartin N. *Healing Conversations: what to say when you don't know what to say.* San Francisco: Jossey-Bass; 2002.

Stone D, Patton B, Heen S. *Difficult Conversations: how to discuss what matters most.* New York: Penguin Books; 1999.

Tamparo CT, Lindh WQ. *Therapeutic Communications for Health Professionals.* 2nd ed. Delmar-Thompson Learning; 2000.

COMMUNICATING IN CRISIS SITUATIONS

Griese NL. *How to Manage Organizational Communications During Crisis.* Atlanta, GA: Anvil Publishers, Inc.; 2001.

Henry RA. *You'd Better Have a Hose if You Want to Put Out the Fire: the complete guide to crisis and risk communication.* Windsor, CA: Gollywobbler Productions; 2000.

Mitroff II, Anagnos G. *Managing Crises Before They Happen: what every executive and manager needs to know about crisis management.* New York: AMACOM; 2001.

Ogrizek M, Guillery J-M. *Communicating in Crisis: a theoretical and practical guide to crisis management.* New York: Aldine de Gruyter; 1999.

Reynolds B, Hunter Galdo J, Sokler L, *et al. Crisis and Emergency Risk Communication.* Atlanta, GA: Centers for Disease Control and Prevention; 2002.

DEALING WITH ORGANIZATIONAL CHANGE

Bridges W. *Managing Transitions: making the most of change.* Cambridge, MA: Perseus Books; 1991.

Kotter JP. *Leading Change.* Boston: Harvard Business School Press; 1996.

Silversin J, Kornacki MJ. *Leading Physicians Through Change: how to achieve and sustain results.* Tampa, FL: American College of Physician Executives; 2000.

COMMUNICATING WITH EMOTIONAL INTELLIGENCE

Bar-On R, Parker JDA. *The Handbook of Emotional Intelligence: theory, development, assessment, and application at home, school, and in the workplace.* San Francisco: Jossey-Bass; 2000.

Cherniss C, Goleman D, editors. *The Emotionally Intelligent Workplace: how to select for, measure, and improve emotional intelligence in individuals, groups, and organizations.* San Francisco: Jossey-Bass; 2001.

Fisher R, Shapiro D. *Beyond Reason: using emotion as you negotiate.* New York: Viking Press; 2005.

Goleman D. *Emotional Intelligence: why it can matter more than IQ.* New York: Bantam Books; 1995.

Goleman D. *Social Intelligence: beyond IQ, beyond emotional intelligence.* New York: Bantam Books; 2006.

Goleman D, Boyatzis R, McKee A. *Primal Leadership: realizing the power of emotional intelligence.* Boston, MA: Harvard Business School Press; 2002.

Hughes M, Terrell JB. *The Emotionally Intelligent Team: understanding and developing the behaviors of success.* San Francisco: Jossey-Bass; 2007.

Keedwell P. *How Sadness Survived: the evolutionary basis of depression.* Abingdon, UK: Radcliffe Publishing; 2008.

Weisinger H. *Emotional Intelligence at Work.* San Francisco: Jossey-Bass; 1998.

3